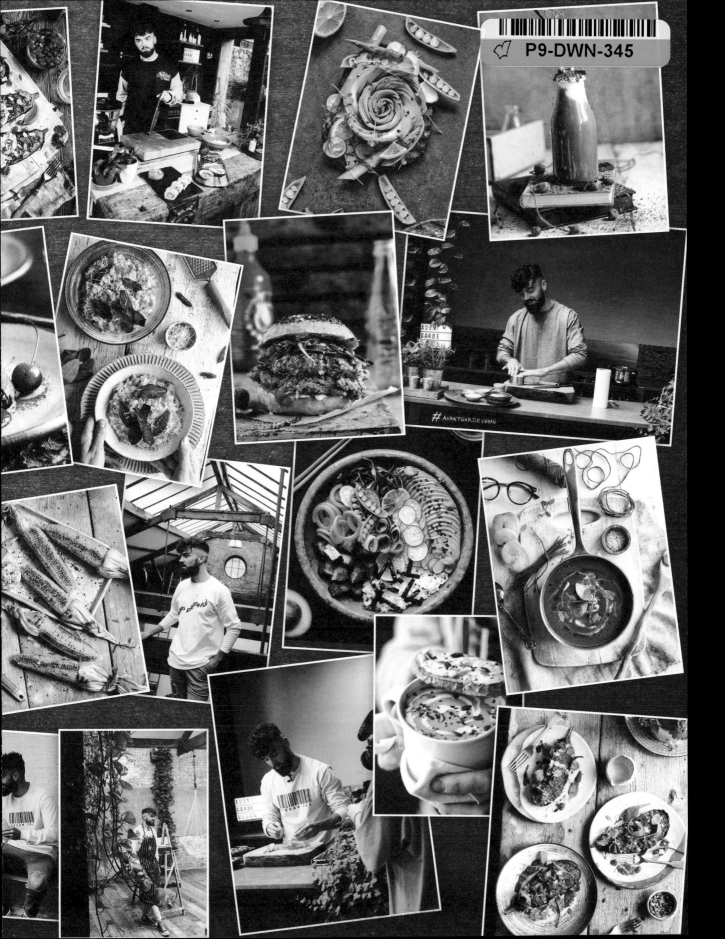

VEGAN

100

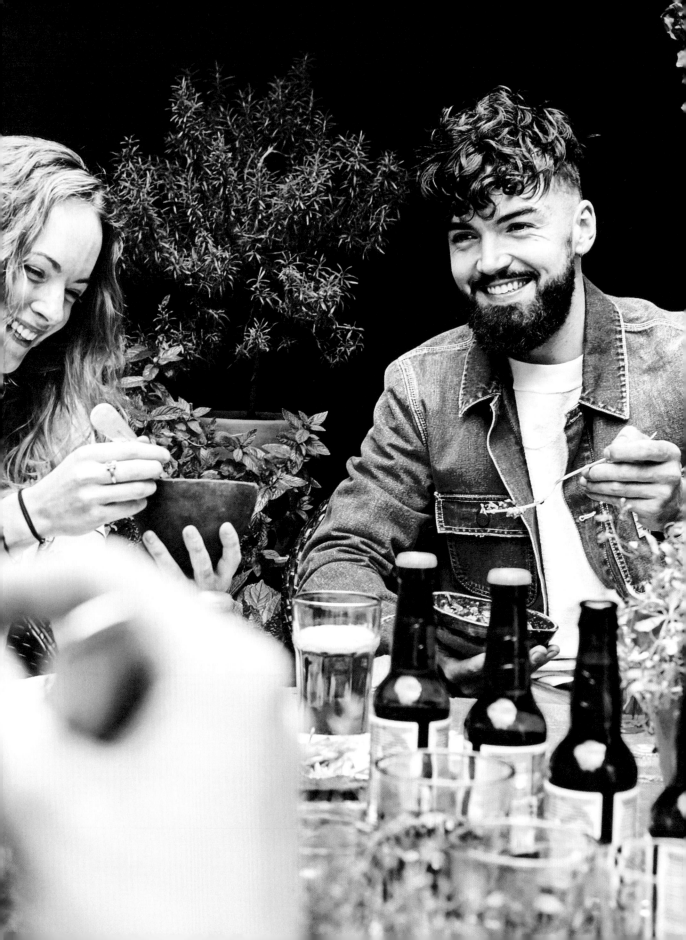

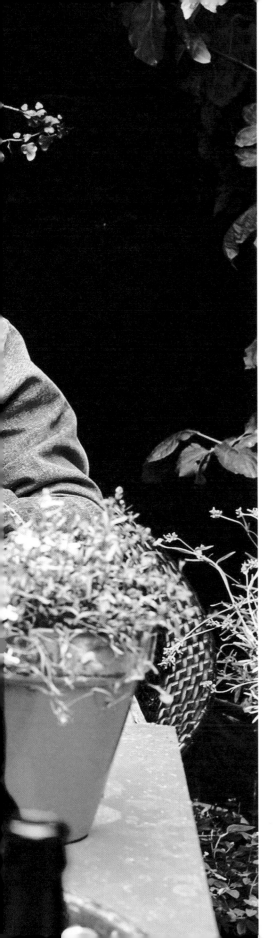

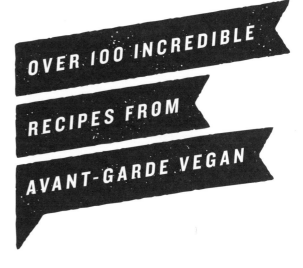

OVER 100 INCREDIBLE

RECIPES FROM

AVANT-GARDE VEGAN

GAZ OAKLEY

**Photography by Simon Smith
and Adam Laycock**

quadrille

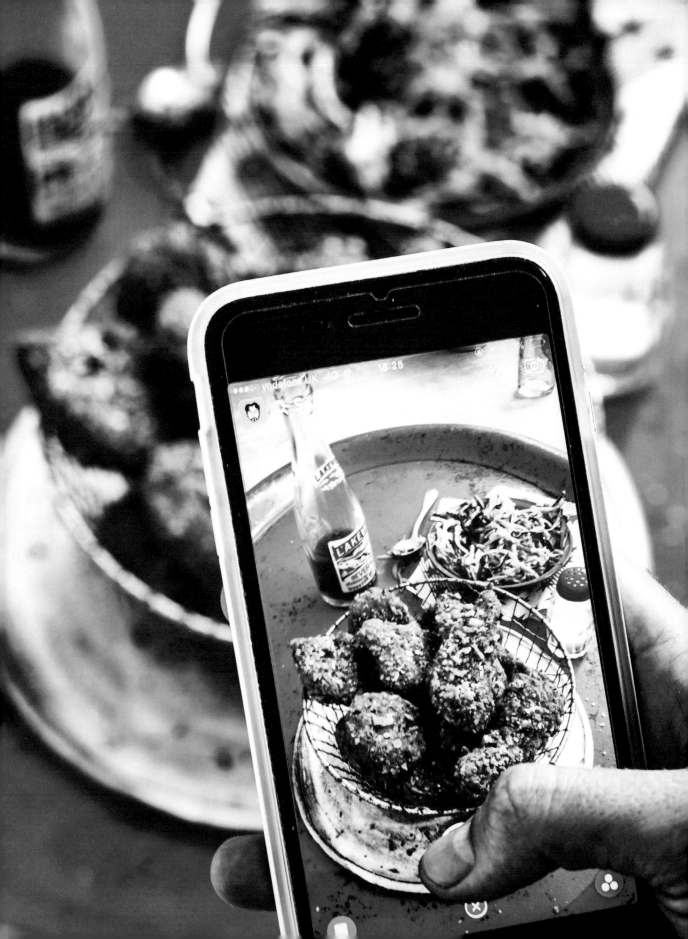

VEGAN 100

INTRODUCTION

Vegan 100 is my debut cookbook – thank you so much for purchasing it!

This has been an absolute pleasure to write. As you may have guessed, I love all things food and cooking. I started Avant-Garde Vegan on Instagram in February 2016, a few months after turning vegan, but my interest in cooking goes back to my childhood. In writing this book, I was determined to include all the recipes I've developed since going vegan. The hardest part of the process was narrowing down the volume of dishes to the best ones that you see here now.

These are the recipes that I wish I had come up with when I first went vegan, for example the really amazing ones that I never would have thought possible when I first started out, like my Seitan Fillet "Steak" Wellington (page 138). I'm hoping this book will help lots of people – all new vegans, everyone who's thinking of going vegan, and seasoned vegans who just want to get a little more adventurous in the kitchen.

One of my biggest concerns in writing the recipes was to make sure that they were all simple enough for anyone to get right. So trust me – although some of the recipes may look long and need more than five ingredients, they are all really doable! And if you have no idea where to begin with vegan ingredients or you're worried about what kind of kitchen equipment you'll need to get the most out of this style of cooking, turn to pages 8 and 9 for a useful list.

Every element in every recipe in this book revolves around bringing big bold flavours to the dish. I have called upon my experience as a chef in professional kitchens to use classic techniques that I guarantee won't fail when you're recreating my food at home.

If you want any more inspiration, or you want to see me in action, please look up my YouTube channel or check out Instagram. No two of my vegan dishes are the same, and you'll be blown away by how amazing they taste.

I really hope you enjoy Vegan 100. Thank you for your support!

Gaz

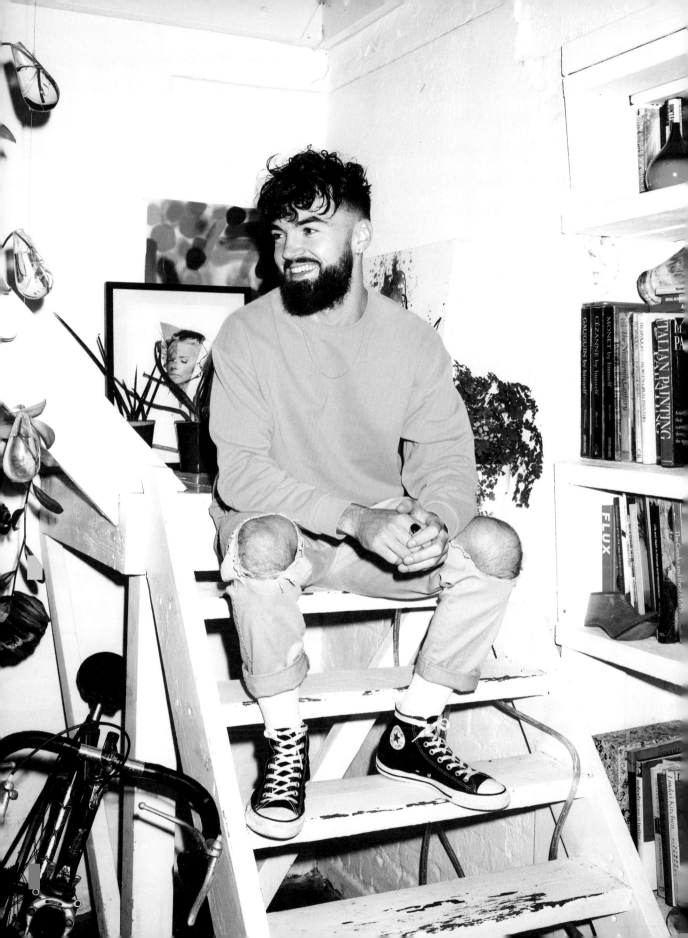

VEGAN INGREDIENTS

AGAR AGAR

Agar agar powder or flakes are a sea-vegetable gelling agent – so basically a vegan gelatine. It's brilliant stuff and can contribute to some amazing dishes!

AGAVE NECTAR

Agave nectar is the sweet nectar extracted from several species of the agave plant, the majority of which are grown in Mexico or South Africa. It is a great natural sweetener. In my recipes, I tend to advise using either agave nectar or maple syrup, as they are very similar in terms of sweetness, however agave is often slightly more affordable.

LECITHIN GRANULES

Made from soy bean oil, these granules give my "Butter" Spread (page 14) a great creaminess. They can be found in all good health food shops, and are good for your kidneys and liver.

LIQUID SMOKE

This handy little flavouring is an optional ingredient in my recipes, but it's absolutely great at creating a smoky flavour.

MISO PASTE

Made from fermented soy beans, this paste has a super-strong umami flavour. You can find it in the Asian section of most supermarkets. It's a staple ingredient in Japanese cooking.

NORI

Nori is made by shredding edible seaweed and then pressing it into thin sheets. It's often used when making sushi.

NUTRITIONAL YEAST

Nutritional yeast is a deactivated yeast. It has a strong flavour that is quite nutty, cheesy and creamy, which makes it the perfect ingredient in my vegan cheese recipes and lots of other recipes where I need a bold flavour.

POMEGRANATE MOLASSES

This is simply pomegranate juice reduced down to form a really sticky, sweet substance.

RAS EL HANOUT

This is a mixture of ground spices. The Arabic name translates as "head of the shop," meaning "the best of the shop."

SEITAN, OR VITAL WHEAT GLUTEN

Wheat gluten, seitan or wheat meat is a food made from gluten – the main protein of wheat. This product has been used in vegetarian recipes for years (Buddhist monks used it as a meat replacement) and it's often used in Asian cookery. I have modernized many ancient recipes to produce some incredible dishes. I love creating dishes with wheat gluten!

TAPIOCA STARCH

Tapioca is extracted from the cassava root. This magic starch gives my cheeses a great stringy, cheese-like texture.

TOFU

Tofu is the first vegan protein people think of. I have some incredible ways to turn this often-boring product into something spectacular. Also known as bean curd, it is cultivated by coagulating soy milk and then pressing the resulting curds into soft, white blocks. Tofu can be soft, firm, or extra firm. I use firm tofu in all the recipes in my book.

USEFUL EQUIPMENT

CHOPPING/CUTTING BOARD

I love my heavy wooden chopping board, and it's adored by many of my YouTube subscribers. I recommend a wooden chopping board, which you should keep as clean as possible and rub olive oil into to keep the wood in good condition after cleaning. Always place a damp cloth underneath your board to stop it from sliding when you're chopping.

GRIDDLE PAN

I love being able to recreate that BBQ/charred flavour in my kitchen by using a griddle pan. Make sure you get a nice heavy cast-iron one which gets brilliantly hot and keeps its heat efficiently.

KNIVES

A set of good chef knives is a must. You should sharpen them before and after using, so you will need a knife steel as well. Check out my knife skills video on YouTube for a few tips on the perfect kitchen knife kit for vegan cooking.

LOOSE-BOTTOM CAKE TINS

I always recommend using a loose-bottom tin when making the cakes or tarts in my book. It makes it a lot easier to remove the bake from the tin and it also makes it look a lot more presentable.

MANDOLINE

This is an essential piece of kit when making recipes like my Aubergine "Bacon" (see page 47) but it also comes in handy when slicing other vegetables extra finely. Make sure you always use it with the guard though!

MEASURING CUPS & KITCHEN SCALES

Most professional chefs don't measure much when they are cooking. Obviously now that I make recipes for a living, I measure everything. For a new cook, I recommend measuring ingredients in cups - it's simple and fast - however, a set of kitchen scales is more accurate for baking.

NON-STICK PANS

Make sure you have a good selection of non-stick frying pans and saucepans in various sizes. Keep them clean and do your best not to scratch them with metal utensils.

POWERFUL BLENDER

One of the most important pieces of equipment in a good vegan kitchen is a powerful blender and lots of my recipes rely on one. I promise that it will be a rally good investment! I recommend a Ninja Kitchen System.

SPATULA

Everything is easier when using a spatula - stirring, scraping, spreading - so make sure you have one! You definitely waste far less of your bake batter or other ingredients when using one.

ESSENTIALS

MILK

Not only is homemade milk much tastier than shop-bought, non-dairy milk, making your own is healthier, more cost-effective and super-easy. I like to know exactly what's in the food I'm eating so I make a couple batches of milk each week; I generally use blanched almonds or cashew nuts.

MAKES 1 litre (1 quart)

125g (1 cup) blanched almonds or cashews OR 100g (1 cup) rolled oats

1 litre (4 cups) ice-cold filtered water

4 Medjool dates, pitted (an optional sweetener, or a little agave nectar or maple syrup to taste)

pinch sea salt

pinch ground cinnamon or grated nutmeg (optional)

Soak the nuts in cold water for at least 8 hours or overnight. I usually soak the nuts before going to bed ready to make the milk in the morning. If you are using oats you do not need to soak them – oat milk is ideal if you need milk quickly!

The next morning, drain away the soaking water, then tip the nuts into a high-speed blender with the cold filtered water and sweetener (if using). Make sure your water is super-cold as the blender will generate some heat which will spoil some of the nutrients if the milk mixture gets warm when blending. Blend until smooth.

Next grab a large jug or container and a milk bag or cheese cloth (or, if you don't have either, a clean tea towel will work perfectly). Secure your cloth over the container and pour the milk mixture through.

Squeeze all the excess liquid out of the mixture, until you've gotten every last speck of liquid out. Then you're done – you should be left with a beautiful fresh batch of the finest milk. Stir in the sea salt, and the cinnamon or nutmeg if using.

Keep the milk in the fridge in a clean covered container for up to 3 days.

Don't just stop at nut and oats. I often make milk with shelled hemp seeds: use the same measurements, don't soak the hemp seeds beforehand, and swap the filtered water for coconut water.

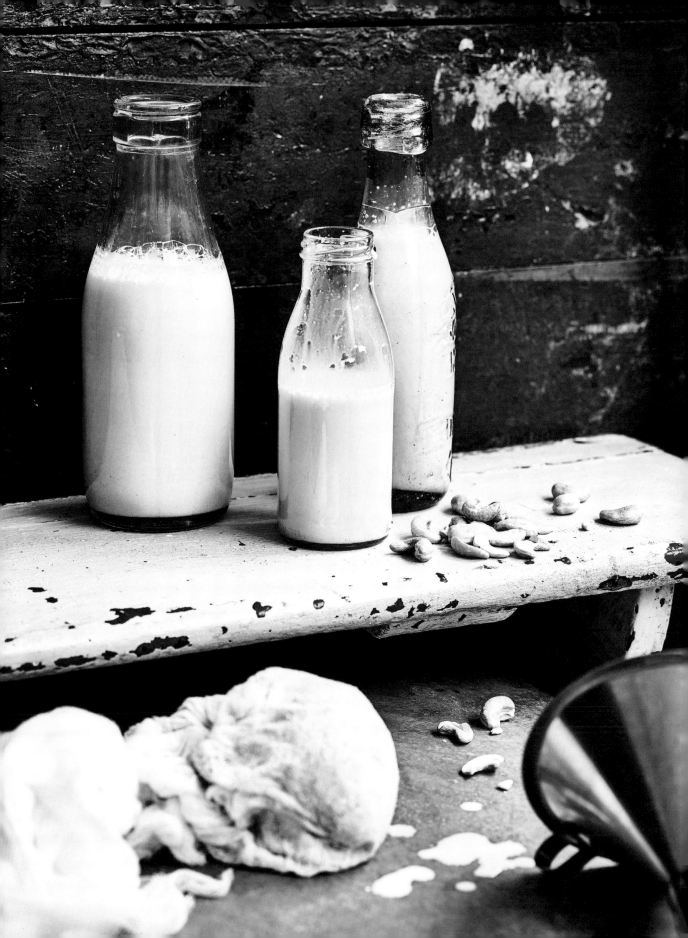

"BUTTER" SPREAD

This spread is great because, like the milk, you know exactly what's going into it. It's a treat to spread on warm toast but also a vital ingredient when making things like pastry. You can freeze the spread, so you can stock up for a while. Rapeseed oil works well here, but experiment with different oils.

MAKES ABOUT 500g (2¼ CUPS)

120ml (½ cup) rapeseed oil

120ml (½ cup) unsweetened soy milk, at room temperature

45g (½ cup) lecithin granules

60ml (¼ cup) unrefined coconut oil, melted

60ml (¼ cup) cacao butter

½ tsp salt

1 tbsp lemon juice

First up, make sure all the ingredients are measured and ready. Set up your high-speed blender, then add all the ingredients to it and blitz for 40 seconds.

You should be left with a beautiful creamy yellow tinted mix, now simply transfer to your chosen containers. I pop some in the freezer and a couple in the fridge. Make sure you cool them quickly to avoid any separation.

The mixture will be quite hard when it first comes out of the fridge, so let it soften slightly before spreading.

"CREAM CHEESE"

There's nothing I love more than this cream cheese spread on a warm bagel with a few cherry tomatoes or avocado on top. Perfect. It's so simple to make and will keep in the fridge for 2-3 days but it's so tasty and indulgent, half the time I've eaten the majority of it before it's even got to the fridge!

MAKES ABOUT 250g (1 CUP)

115g ($^3/_4$ cup) raw cashew nuts

120ml ($^1/_2$ cup) cashew milk

2 tbsp nutritional yeast flakes

1 tbsp lemon juice

pinch sea salt and white pepper

$^1/_4$ tsp dried onion granules

First up, "quick soak" the nuts: simply pop them in a heatproof container and pour over boiling water. Leave for around 20 minutes to soften while you measure out the other ingredients.

Drain the water from the nuts and tip them into a high-speed blender. Add the rest of the ingredients and blend for 15 seconds. You will probably need to scrape down the sides and give everything a little stir, then blend again until smooth.

The smoother this cheese is the better, so add a little more milk if you think it needs it.

Once smooth, spoon the mixture into a lidded container and keep refrigerated.

SMOKED PAPRIKA & SAGE "CHEESE"

I absolutely love a smoky flavour, but you can leave out the smoked paprika if you want your cheese to have a more neutral flavour. The agar agar helps set it perfectly – the great thing about this cheese is that you can slice it and it even melts when you heat it up.

MAKES 4 LITTLE "CHEESES"

a little coconut oil, for greasing

90g ($^3/_4$ cup) blanched almonds or cashews

240ml (1 cup) soy milk

2 tbsp tapioca starch

2 tbsp nutritional yeast

1 tsp sweet smoked paprika, plus extra to garnish

1 tsp dried sage, plus extra to garnish

1 tbsp lemon juice

1 tbsp agar agar powder

pinch sea salt and white pepper

Grease 4 ramekins with a little coconut oil.

"Quick soak" the nuts: simply pop them in a heatproof container and pour over boiling water. Leave for around 20 minutes to soften while you measure out the other ingredients.

Once the nuts have softened, drain and add them to a high-speed blender with all the other ingredients. Blend until you have a super-smooth, creamy mixture.

Scrape the mixture into a saucepan. Using a spatula, stir the mixture over a low heat until it starts to thicken. Continue to stir constantly until the mixture is really thick and has a melted cheese-like consistency. It's essential that you stir the mixture continuously as it can easily catch on the bottom which totally spoils the flavour, so try not to have any distractions.

Remove the pan from the heat and pour the mixture into your prepared containers and chill in the fridge for 2 hours, or until set through. This cheese will keep for 4–5 days in the fridge.

To serve, remove the cheese from the container, sprinkle over some sage and paprika, slice and enjoy!

"CRÈME FRAÎCHE"

This is the perfect topping for nachos, chilli, or any dish that needs a little cooling down.

MAKES ABOUT 5 SERVINGS

75g (½ cup) raw cashew nuts

2 tbsp lemon juice

pinch salt and white pepper

110ml (½ cup) filtered water

"Quick soak" the nuts: simply pop them in a heatproof container and pour over boiling water. Leave for around 20 minutes to soften while you measure out the other ingredients.

Once the nuts have softened, drain and add them to a high-speed blender with the rest of the ingredients. Simply blitz everything until smooth, then serve or store in the fridge for 3–4 days.

MELTABLE "MOZZARELLA"

This recipe took a lot of experimenting to get right, but I was so impressed when I cracked it – it's the most incredible vegan mozzarella and the perfect cheese for topping pizzas or filling quesadillas. You can form the mix into balls but I prefer to keep it in a sealed container and spoon it on as and when I need it.

MAKES ABOUT 5 SERVINGS

75g ($^1/_2$ cup) raw cashew nuts

240ml (1 cup) cold Milk (see page 12)

4 tbsp tapioca starch

2 tbsp nutritional yeast

$^1/_4$ tsp dried onion powder

1 tsp white miso

1 tsp lemon juice

pinch sea salt and white pepper

$^1/_4$ tsp garlic powder

First, "quick soak" the nuts: simply pop them in a heatproof container and pour over boiling water. Leave for around 20 minutes to soften while you measure out the other ingredients.

Once the nuts have softened, drain and add them to a high-speed blender with all the other ingredients. Blend on full speed until you have a smooth mixture. I know it doesn't look anything like mozzarella now, but bear with it!

Scrape the cheese mixture into a non-stick saucepan, arm yourself with a spatula and start stirring over a medium heat. Be patient – you will be stirring for around 8–10 minutes. Stir until it is super-thick and starts to come away from the sides of the saucepan.

Once it's thick and cheese-like, remove from the heat. Serve straight away or place in a sealed container and store in the fridge for up to 3 days.

"Mozzarella"

"Cream Cheese"

Smoked Paprika & Sage "Cheese"

BASIC HOMEMADE PASTA

Making your own pasta feels so rewarding. It's one of the first skills I learned when I started cooking.
This recipe produces a heavenly light pasta which can be made into raviolis and so much more.

MAKES 4 SERVINGS

180g (1½ cups) 00 white flour

60g (½ cup) Kamut flour

pinch sea salt

4 tbsp extra virgin olive oil

160ml (⅔ cup) cold water

Sift the flours and salt into a large bowl. Make a well in the centre and add the olive oil and half of the water.

Stir with your fingers or a cutlery knife. Add enough of the remaining water to bring everything together into a ball.

Lightly knead the dough for a minute or so, wrap in cling film (plastic wrap) and pop the pasta dough in the fridge to rest for 15 minutes. In the meantime, set up your pasta machine.

Cut the dough into 3, then roll to your desired thickness, making sure you have floured the machine and pasta. You can roll your pasta with a rolling pin, but I really recommend getting a pasta machine. You will enjoy making pasta so much more!

Cut and shape into the pasta of your choice. This will keep in the fridge for up to 2 days.

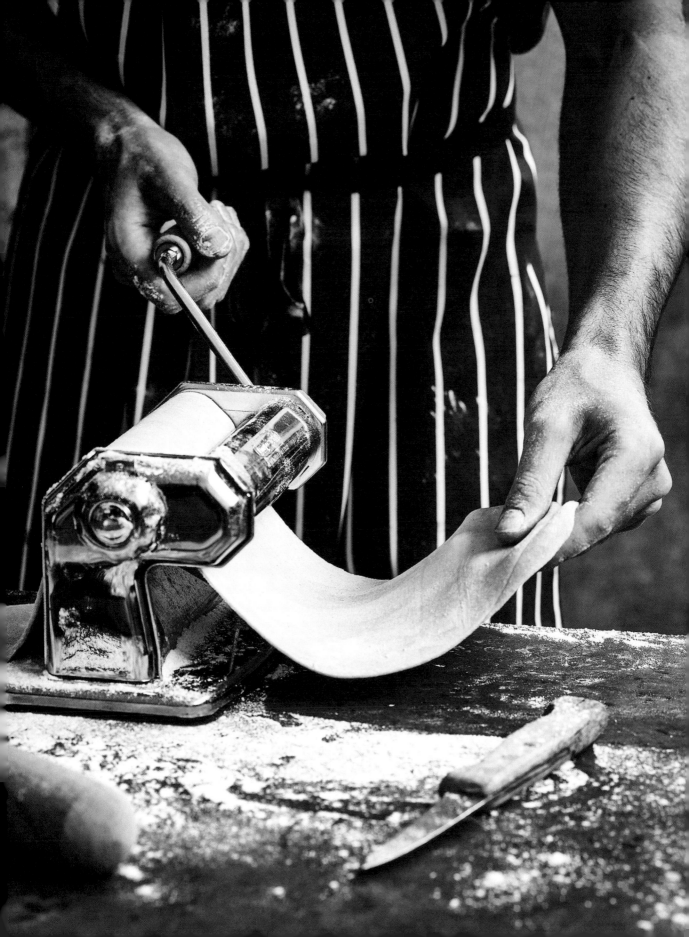

CHOCOLATE NOT-ELLA HAZELNUT SPREAD

It was great to see the delight on my mum's face when she first tasted this after missing Nutella. It's identical in flavour; in fact it is a little bit delightful, if I do say so myself, and you know exactly what's gone into it! This also makes an incredible chocolate sauce if you heat a tablespoon with half a cup of almond milk.

MAKES A 227-g (8-oz) JAR

140g (1 cup) raw hazelnuts

1 tsp vanilla extract

25g (1/4 cup) organic cocoa powder

4 tbsp agave nectar or maple syrup

pinch sea salt

2 tbsp melted coconut oil

240ml (1 cup) milk (I use hazelnut Milk; see page 12)

Simply throw everything into a high-speed blender and blend for 20 seconds. Open it and check it as you may have to scrape the sides and give it a little mix, then blend for a further 20 seconds, or until it's totally smooth.

Pop into a sterilized 227-g (8-oz) jar or container and into the fridge where it will keep for up to 4 days.

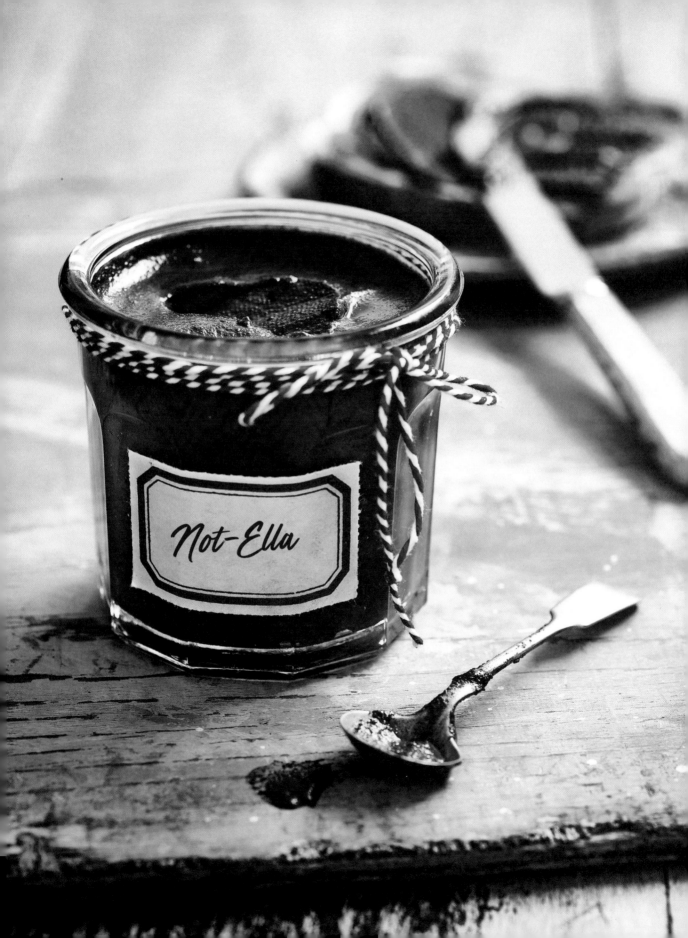

CREAMY "MAYONNAISE"

I couldn't not put this recipe in my book for you guys; the taste will leave you wondering why mayonnaise was ever made with eggs!

MAKES A 227-g (8-oz) JAR

120ml (½ cup)
unsweetened soy milk

1 tsp apple cider vinegar

1 tsp lemon juice

240ml (1 cup) rapeseed oil

pinch sea salt and white pepper

I strongly recommend using a hand stick blender for this recipe. Simply combine the milk, vinegar and lemon juice in a tall jug. Now, whilst blending, gradually drizzle in the oil. Keep blending until you've added all the oil and you have a creamy mayo-like consistency. Add seasoning to taste.

This mayonnaise can be stored in sealed containers in the fridge for around a week.

BBQ SAUCE

This smoky sauce complements my Chilli Dogs on page 108 so well. It also works as a pretty decent marinade for things like tofu and tempeh. It has a rich hickory-style taste thanks to some smoked paprika and liquid smoke.

MAKES 200ml (¾ CUP)

120ml (½ cup) Classic Tomato Ketchup (see opposite)

2 tsp maple syrup

2 tbsp tamari or soy sauce

1 tbsp white wine vinegar

¼ tsp cayenne pepper

¼ tsp smoked paprika

¼ tsp garlic powder

¼ tsp mustard powder

1–2 drops of liquid smoke

Add all the ingredients to a heavy-based saucepan and stir everything together over a low heat. All you really want to do is let the flavours mingle together. Heat for around 4 minutes.

Remove from the heat, cool for a minute or so, then pour into sterilized jars or containers and store in the fridge. It will keep for up to 1 week.

ESSENTIALS

HOT PINK BEETROOT KETCHUP

This recipe has no tomatoes in sight. The natural sweetness and earthy, rich flavour of beetroots make them the perfect ingredient for ketchup, and the pink colour just makes it even more spectacular.

MAKES ABOUT 200ml (³/₄ CUP)

500g (3 cups) cubed, cooked red beetroot (beet)

120ml (¹/₂ cup) white wine vinegar

240ml (1 cup) water

5 tbsp organic unrefined caster (superfine) sugar

1 bay leaf

2 shallots, finely chopped

pinch sea salt and cracked black pepper

Heat all the ingredients in a heavy-based saucepan over a medium heat and allow to simmer for around 10 minutes, or until the shallots are cooked and the liquid has slightly thickened.

Remove from the heat and let the mixture cool slightly before removing the bay leaf. Then tip into a blender and blend until super-smooth; it should be bright pink and have that glossy ketchup look.

Carefully pour into sterilized jars or containers then pop into the fridge to chill. Serve and use like ketchup. I generally keep the ketchup for no longer than 3 weeks.

CLASSIC TOMATO KETCHUP

Classic ketchup! I made a ketchup on YouTube using fresh tomatoes, but this one uses tomato puree so you will be left with a more traditional-style ketchup – the perfect mix of sweet, spice and, of course, tanginess.

MAKES 200ml (³/₄ CUP)

110g (¹/₂ cup) organic tomato puree

3 tbsp white wine vinegar

65g (¹/₃ cup) unrefined caster (superfine) sugar

240ml (1 cup) water

¹/₂ tsp sea salt

¹/₂ tsp ground black pepper

¹/₄ tsp garlic powder

¹/₄ tsp onion powder

¹/₄ tsp cayenne pepper

Simply combine all the ingredients in a small non-stick saucepan. Cook over a medium heat, stirring often, until all the sugar has dissolved and the flavours are starting to mingle.

Cook for a further 2 minutes, then carefully pour into sterilized bottles or containers and chill.

Feel free to experiment with different flavours – smoky paprika works really well.

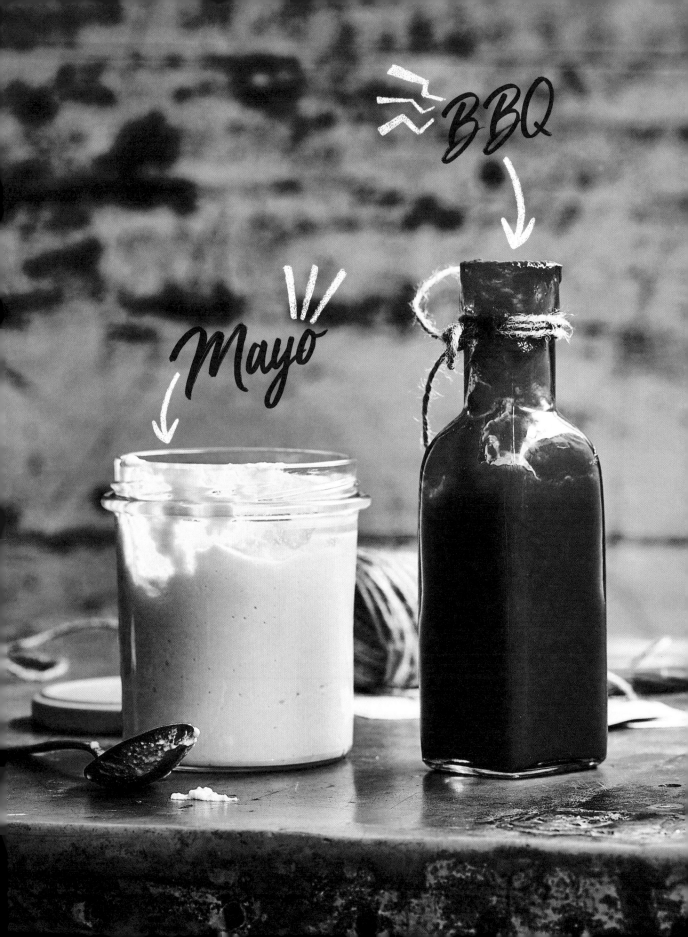

Mayo

BBQ

Beetroot
Ketchup

Classic
Ketchup

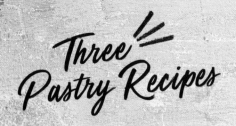

SAVOURY SHORTCRUST PASTRY

**This is the perfect crust for pies, hot pots and so much more.
Just a few ingredients make this excellent "works every time" pastry.**

**MAKES ENOUGH TO
LINE A 23-cm (9-inch)
PIE, TOP & BOTTOM**

125g (1 cup) "Butter" Spread
(see page 14) or vegan margarine

375g (3 cups) plain
(all-purpose) flour

pinch salt

2 tbsp almond Milk (see page 12)

Place all the ingredients except
the milk in a large mixing bowl. Rub
the butter into the flour and salt
with your fingertips until the mix
resembles breadcrumbs.

Pour in enough milk to bring the
dough together into a ball and pick
up all the bits from the bowl. Give
the dough a slight knead for

about 2 minutes and that's it,
pastry done!

I divide mine into 3, wrap it in cling
film (plastic wrap), then pop it in
the fridge or freezer depending
on when I'm using it. This pastry
can be frozen for up to 2 months.
Defrost fully before using.

SWEET PASTRY

This is my go-to recipe for all desserts that require pastry. It's so simple to make and if you are feeling lazy you can actually throw everything into a blender to mix without getting your hands messy. I make batches and store them in the freezer.

**MAKES ENOUGH TO
LINE A 23-cm (9-inch)
PIE, TOP & BOTTOM**

125g (1 cup) "Butter" Spread
(see page 14) or vegan margarine

250g (2 cups) plain
(all-purpose) flour

125g (1 cup) icing
(confectioner's) sugar

pinch salt

pinch ground cinnamon

2 tbsp almond Milk (see page 12)

Place all the ingredients except the milk in a large mixing bowl. Rub the butter into the dry ingredients with your fingertips until the mixture resembles breadcrumbs.

Pour in enough milk to bring the dough together into a ball and pick up all the bits from the bowl. Give it a slight knead for 2 minutes and that's it; sweet pastry done.

I portion mine up into 3, wrap in cling film (plastic wrap), then pop into the fridge for 2 days or freezer for up to 2 months depending on when I'm using it. Check out my Sweet Talking chapter on page 182 for some mouthwatering pastry desserts.

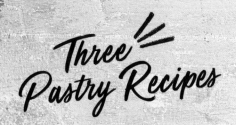

ROUGH PUFF PASTRY

It's actually uncommon to see a non-vegan chef making their own homemade puff pastry these days but it was one of the first things I learned to make when I became a chef at 15. This rough vegan version is much simpler to make – you will wow your friends when you tell them you have made this delightful flaky pastry.

MAKES ENOUGH TO LINE A 23-cm (9-inch) PIE, TOP & BOTTOM

250g (2 cups) plain (all-purpose) flour

pinch salt

250g (2 cups) "Butter" Spread (see page 14), at room temperature but not soft

5 tbsp water

Sift the flour and salt into a large bowl. Add the butter in small chunks and lightly rub the butter in. You want to still see the butter pieces so don't over-rub. Make a well in the centre and pour in enough water to form into a dough.

Cover the bowl and place it in the fridge to rest for around 15 minutes.

Lightly flour your clean work surface, then knead the pastry into a rectangle shape. Roll the dough in one direction until it's approximately 3 times longer than the original rectangle – around

20 x 50cm (8 x 20 inches) will do – keeping the edges nice and square.

Fold the top end into the centre, then the other end over the top. Turn the pastry 90 degrees, then repeat the process. I do this 3 times, turning 90 degrees between each roll and fold.

Chill the pastry for 20 minutes before rolling out and cooking. (Or you can store in the fridge for 2 days or freeze for up to 2 months until you want to use it.)

VEGETABLE STOCK

**A good stock is essential for any budding home cook.
Feel free to just use my recipe as a guide and use whatever vegetables you
have in your fridge – pack as much flavour into it as you can.**

MAKES ABOUT 1 litre (1 quart)

1 white onion

$\frac{1}{2}$ leek

2 garlic cloves

1 carrot

1 stick of celery

handful of chestnut mushrooms

1 tbsp extra virgin olive oil

handful of chopped
parsley and stalks

1 tsp salt

1 tsp cracked black pepper

Chop the vegetables and
mushrooms into small pieces.

Heat a large heavy-based
saucepan over a medium heat
and add the olive oil. Add all the
vegetables, herbs and mushrooms
to the pan and sweat them for
around 3 minutes, so they start
releasing their flavours.

Add the salt and pepper followed
by enough water to cover the
vegetables. Allow to simmer for
15 minutes.

Pour the stock mixture through
a sieve and discard the vegetable
pieces or keep for another use.
The liquid stock is ready to
be used.

It can be stored in the fridge for up
to 3 days; I freeze mine in batches
to use as and when.

EGG REPLACEMENT

This is key in any vegan kitchen as it really helps bind ingredients in many of my recipes. Chia seeds expand when left to soak in liquid and they become gelatinous, which makes them a great swap for eggs in recipes.

MAKES ABOUT 1 HEAPED tbsp OR THE EQUIVALENT OF 1 EGG

5 tbsp white chia seeds

filtered water

Blitz the chia seeds in a high-speed blender until ground. For every 1 tbsp ground seeds, add 3 tbsp filtered cold water and mix well.

Place the mixture into a sealed container and store in the fridge for up to 2 weeks. Use as and when. I use 1 heaped tbsp of the mixture for 1 egg.

PEANUT & ALMOND BUTTER

Once you make this you will never buy shop-bought nut butters again! It is so simple to make and with just a few ingredients you can achieve that creamy, nutty spread. I like my nut butter to have a roasted flavour but if you prefer to keep it raw, skip the roasting step.

MAKES A 227-g (8-oz) JAR

125g (1 cup) raw shelled and skinned peanuts

125g (1 cup) blanched almonds

1 tbsp peanut oil (or a flavourless oil of your choice)

pinch sea salt

1 tbsp agave nectar or maple syrup (optional)

Line a baking tray with baking parchment and preheat the oven to 180°C (350°F). Spread the peanuts and almonds out on the tray and roast in the oven for 8 minutes, or until golden brown.

Tip the nuts into a high-speed blender and have a spatula to hand. Blend the nuts into a fine crumb-like consistency. This will take a couple minutes of stopping and starting when you will have to scrape the nuts from the side of the blender.

Once you have fine crumbs they will start to clump together and all you need to do is add the oil, salt and agave or maple syrup (if using). Give it one final mix and you should be left with creamy peanut and almond butter. Easy as that!

Try adding 1 tbsp cacao powder and 1 tsp vanilla for a sweet twist.

BREAKFAST & BRUNCH

Sage & Apple
Breakfast Sausages

Super Bean Sausages

Paprika Baked Beans

Scrambled Tofu with
Spinach & Cherry Tomatoes

Smashed Avo

Smoky Tempeh "Bacon"

Aubergine "Bacon"

Maple "Pumpkin Pie" Pancakes

Tropical Chia Seed Pudding

Fruity Quinoa Salad

Gaz's Granola with
Caramelized Cherries

Moroccan Chickpea
"Omelette"

SAGE & APPLE BREAKFAST SAUSAGES

Here is the ultimate vegan sausage made with wheat gluten or, as we vegans call it, seitan. Follow my recipe and you will end up with a juicy, surprisingly meaty sausage which, as I know from personal experience, I missed a lot when I first went vegan. I recommend making these sausages the day before using; you can even freeze them.

MAKES 8

Wet ingredients:

180ml ($^3/_4$ cup) hot Vegetable Stock (see page 31)

3 tbsp dried porcini mushrooms

a little coconut oil

1 red onion, evenly chopped

2 garlic cloves, crushed

1 medium sweet apple, peeled and cut into 1-cm ($^1/_2$-inch) cubes

120ml ($^1/_2$ cup) apple juice

3 tbsp tomato puree

1 tbsp soy sauce

1 tbsp white miso paste

$^1/_2$ tsp sea salt

$^1/_2$ tsp cracked black pepper

$^1/_4$ tsp cayenne pepper

1 tbsp dried sage

1 tsp fennel seeds

light olive oil, for oiling

Dry ingredients:

270g ($2^1/_3$ cups) seitan (vital wheat gluten)

50g ($^1/_2$ cup) chickpea (gram) flour

Mix the hot vegetable stock with the porcini and set aside for 5 minutes to allow the porcini to rehydrate.

Preheat a non-stick saucepan and add a touch of coconut oil. When the pan is hot, add the onion, garlic and apple cubes. Lower the heat and allow them to soften and lightly caramelize for around 2 minutes, stirring often. After 2 minutes add the apple juice and deglaze the pan. Cook for a further 2 minutes, or until the apple has softened.

Remove the pan from the heat and tip the mix into a blender cup with the remaining wet ingredients, plus the mushroom and stock mixture. Let the mixture sit for 5 minutes to cool slightly while you put the seitan and chickpea flour in a large mixing bowl.

Blitz the wet mixture in the blender until smooth. Pour the wet mixture into the dry ingredients and quickly stir with a spatula until everything is well combined.

You will need to use your hands at this point to knead the mixture together. Knead for around 10 minutes either in the bowl or on a clean surface. Your dough will be quite wet so feel free to put a light sprinkling of chickpea flour on the surface. The firmer you are when kneading, the more of a bite/meat-like texture your sausages will have when cooked, so be firm!

Once kneaded, divide the dough into approximately 8 pieces; I weigh each piece to make sure all my sausages are a similar size. Aim for around 110g (4oz) per sausage.

Heat a large saucepan half-full of water, bring it to the boil, then turn the heat down low, so that the water is at a rolling simmer.

Prepare 8 pieces of foil, shiny side up, approximately 25cm (10 inches) long. Alternatively, if you don't like using foil, use greaseproof baking paper instead.

[Continued on page 38...]

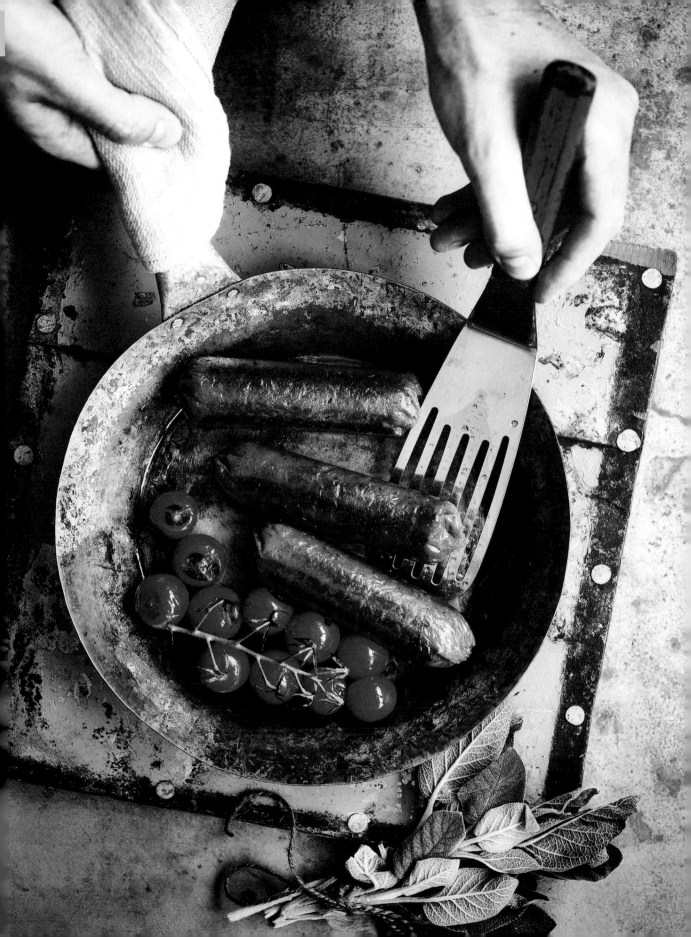

SAGE & APPLE BREAKFAST SAUSAGES (CONT.)

Add a little bit of light olive oil to the shiny side. Individually roll each piece of dough into a sausage shape with your hands before rolling up in the foil. Twist each end and set aside. Do this for the rest of the dough pieces, then wrap each sausage tightly in cling film (plastic wrap).

Lower the sausages into the saucepan of simmering water, pop the lid on and cook for 50 minutes, giving them a little stir every now and then. Don't let them boil – keep a constant, slow simmer.

After the 50 minutes, the sausages should be firm to the touch. Lift one out with a slotted spoon to check. Be careful because they will be very hot! If they are still soft pop them back in the water to cook for a further 10 minutes. Once the sausages are cooked and cool enough to handle, remove the wrapping.

Sauté them lightly in oil, or bake in an oven at 180°C (350°F), for about 10 minutes or until golden.

SUPER BEAN SAUSAGES

This is my gluten-free sausage option which is packed full of some stunning flavours and healthy beans. They're a great sausage for any time of the day but I love them for brunch.

MAKES 7

1 tbsp coconut oil

$\frac{1}{2}$ red onion, finely chopped

1 garlic clove, crushed

$\frac{1}{2}$ red (bell) pepper, deseeded and finely chopped

5 sun-dried tomatoes, finely chopped

25g ($\frac{1}{4}$ cup) finely chopped chestnut mushrooms

$\frac{1}{4}$ tsp fennel seeds, toasted and ground

$\frac{1}{4}$ tsp cayenne pepper

$\frac{1}{4}$ tsp paprika

$\frac{1}{4}$ tsp dried oregano

1 x 400-g (14-oz) can black beans, drained and rinsed

1 x 400-g (14-oz) can kidney beans, drained and rinsed

1 tbsp tomato puree

2 tsp nutritional yeast

1 tbsp balsamic vinegar

5 tbsp buckwheat flour

2 tbsp pine nuts, crushed

$\frac{1}{4}$ tsp cracked black pepper

$\frac{1}{4}$ tsp sea salt

Preheat a non-stick frying pan over a medium heat. Add the coconut oil, followed by the onion, garlic, pepper, sun-dried tomatoes, mushrooms, spices and oregano.

Sauté for 2-3 minutes, stirring often, until everything has softened. Set aside.

Lightly mash the black beans and kidney beans in a large bowl using a potato masher until they are mixed together. Add the contents of the frying pan, followed by the tomato puree, yeast, vinegar, buckwheat flour, pine nuts and seasoning. Mix everything together with a spatula until well incorporated. If your mix is still quite wet add slightly more flour.

Prepare 7 pieces of baking paper and foil around 25cm (10 inches) long. Divide the mixture into 7, then shape into rough sausage shapes

with your hands. Roll the sausage shapes individually in baking paper first, twisting the ends, then wrap in the foil and twist the ends again. Once all the sausages are rolled up in foil, roll each one tightly in cling film (plastic wrap).

Bring a large pan of water to the boil, reduce to a simmer and lower in the sausages. Lightly poach the sausages for 15 minutes – don't let the water boil.

After 15 minutes turn the heat off and leave the sausages in the water for around 10 minutes before removing them and allowing to cool. When they're cool enough to handle, carefully remove the wrapping.

Sauté in a little coconut oil or bake in the oven at 180°C (350°F) for 10 minutes or until nicely golden.

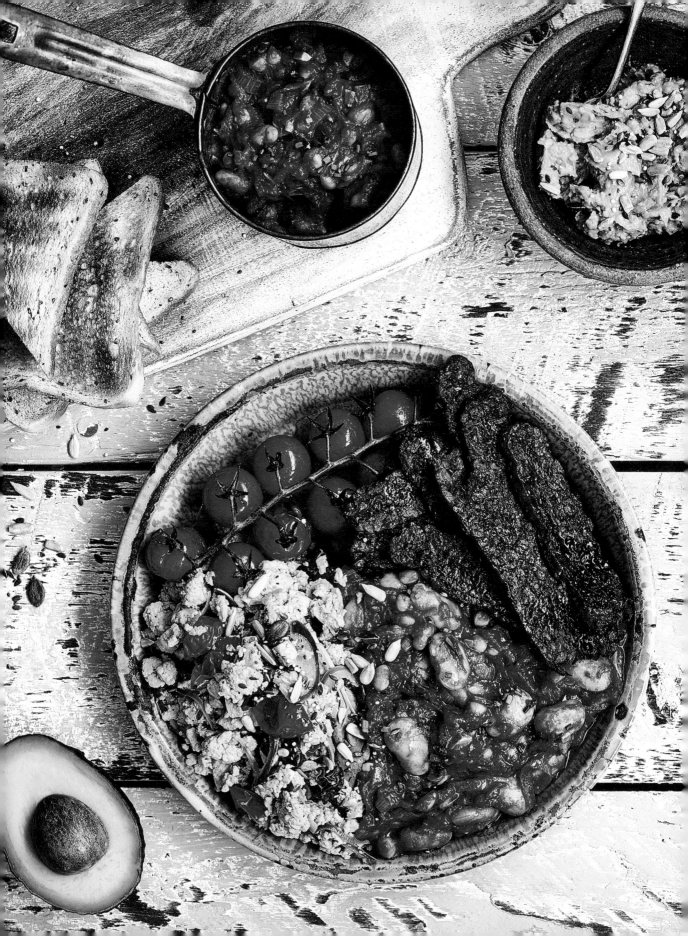

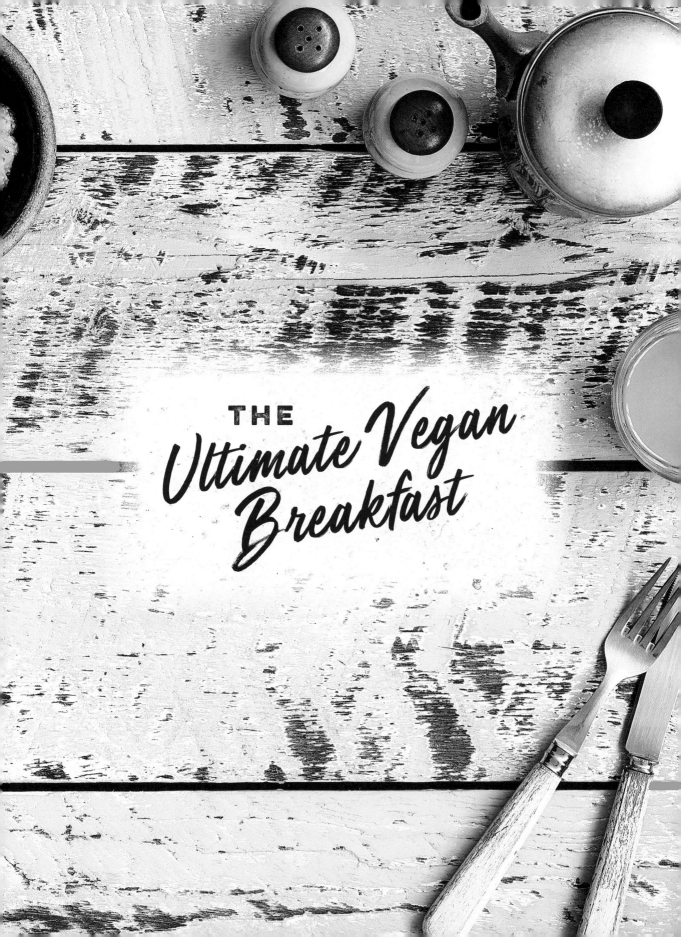

THE
Ultimate Vegan Breakfast

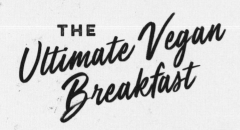

PAPRIKA BAKED BEANS

This is my little twist on classic baked beans with rich, tangy goodness. They are the perfect accompaniment to any breakfast.

SERVES 4

1 tbsp olive oil

2 shallots, finely chopped

1 garlic clove, crushed

1 tsp smoked paprika

pinch sea salt and pepper

1 x 400-g (14-oz) can chopped tomatoes

2 tbsp unrefined caster (granulated) sugar

1 tbsp white wine vinegar

200g (1 cup) canned butter beans

200g (1 cup) canned haricot beans

1 tbsp finely chopped flat leaf parsley

Heat the olive oil in a non-stick saucepan and sweat the shallots and garlic for approximately 2 minutes, stirring often to avoid anything burning. Add the paprika and seasoning, then cook for 1 minute more.

Turn the heat right down, then add the tomatoes, sugar and white wine vinegar. Bring this to a simmer, then add the cooked beans, stirring to combine.

Cook for 3–4 minutes, stirring often. Check for seasoning, then serve with a sprinkling of parsley.

SCRAMBLED TOFU WITH SPINACH & CHERRY TOMATOES

Scrambled tofu is the best start to a day for me – it is the perfect, and even tastier, equivalent to scrambled eggs. It is an amazing source of protein, iron and calcium. The optional Kala Namak (Indian black salt) adds a sulphuric, egg-like taste.

SERVES 4

1 tbsp coconut oil

1 medium red onion, finely chopped

1 x 400-g (14-oz) block of firm tofu, drained

1 tsp ground turmeric

$\frac{1}{4}$ tsp cayenne pepper

2 tbsp nutritional yeast

$\frac{1}{4}$ cup almond Milk (see page 12)

handful of fresh baby spinach

150g (1 cup) cherry tomatoes, halved

pinch Kala Namak (optional)

pinch sea salt and cracked black pepper

2 tbsp mixed seeds, to serve

Preheat a large non-stick frying pan over a medium heat and add the coconut oil followed by the chopped onion. Sweat the onion until soft, stirring often.

While the onion is cooking, drain the excess water from the tofu. Using kitchen paper, press on the block, absorbing the water. You will never remove all the water, but remove as much as you can.

When the onions are soft, crumble the tofu using your hands into the frying pan. Give it a stir and sauté for 2 minutes.

Add the turmeric, cayenne, yeast and almond milk. Turn the heat down and stir for 2 minutes. It should really start to resemble scrambled eggs at this point.

Turn up the heat and quickly add the spinach and tomatoes, stirring for 1 minute or until the spinach has wilted. Season with Kala Namak, if using, sea salt, and pepper to taste.

Serve with a sprinkling of mixed seeds.

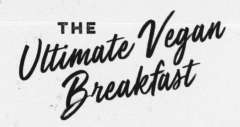

THE *Ultimate Vegan Breakfast*

SMASHED AVO

This is the ideal dish to make with over-ripe avocados – there's nothing better served on a warm bagel. Achieving this avo-goodness couldn't be simpler; the other ingredients totally transform the flavour of the avocado. This adds a real freshness to my cooked breakfast.

SERVES 4

2 very ripe avocados, peeled and de-stoned

juice of ½ lime

pinch sea salt and cracked black pepper

1 tbsp chopped fresh chives

¼ tsp dried chilli flakes (optional)

Throw the avocado flesh into a bowl and give it a good old mash. Stir in the rest of the ingredients. Check for seasoning.

The lime not only seasons the avocado, it keeps the colour green, so in theory you can make this a couple of hours in advance. However, it is best eaten straight away.

SMOKY TEMPEH "BACON"

Tempeh isn't the most exciting-tasting ingredient, but when you give it a "bacony" flavour make-over it's incredible. It is also full of some great vitamins and nutrients. I cook my tempeh bacon in a broth first to guarantee the incredible smoky flavours.

SERVES 4

1 x 200-g (7-oz) block of tempeh

For the broth:

960ml (4 cups) Vegetable Stock (see page 31)

1 tbsp soy sauce (or use tamari for gluten-free)

5 tbsp maple syrup

1 tbsp balsamic vinegar

1 tbsp liquid smoke

1 tbsp brown rice miso

1 tsp smoked paprika

1 tsp dried sage

1 bay leaf

First up we need to make a broth. Add all the broth ingredients to a large, lidded saucepan and give it a good old mix. Pop the saucepan on the stove with a lid on and bring the broth to a rolling simmer. This activates all the flavours.

Meanwhile, slice the tempeh into approximately 3–4-mm ($\frac{1}{8}$-inch) thick slices, then carefully place the tempeh slices into the broth.

Gently simmer the tempeh in the broth for around 20 minutes, with the lid on, stirring now and then.

After 20 minutes, some of the broth should have been absorbed by the tempeh and it should smell beautiful and smoky.

Very carefully remove the tempeh slices from the pan and place them on a baking tray lined with greaseproof paper. Preheat your grill (broiler).

Turn the heat up under the broth and boil until it reduces right down to almost a glaze-like consistency. This should take around 3–5 minutes, depending on how much broth was absorbed by the tempeh.

When reduced, brush the glaze over the tempeh slices, then place the tray under the grill for 12 minutes.

Serve the tempeh bacon with your breakfast or use as the perfect sandwich filler.

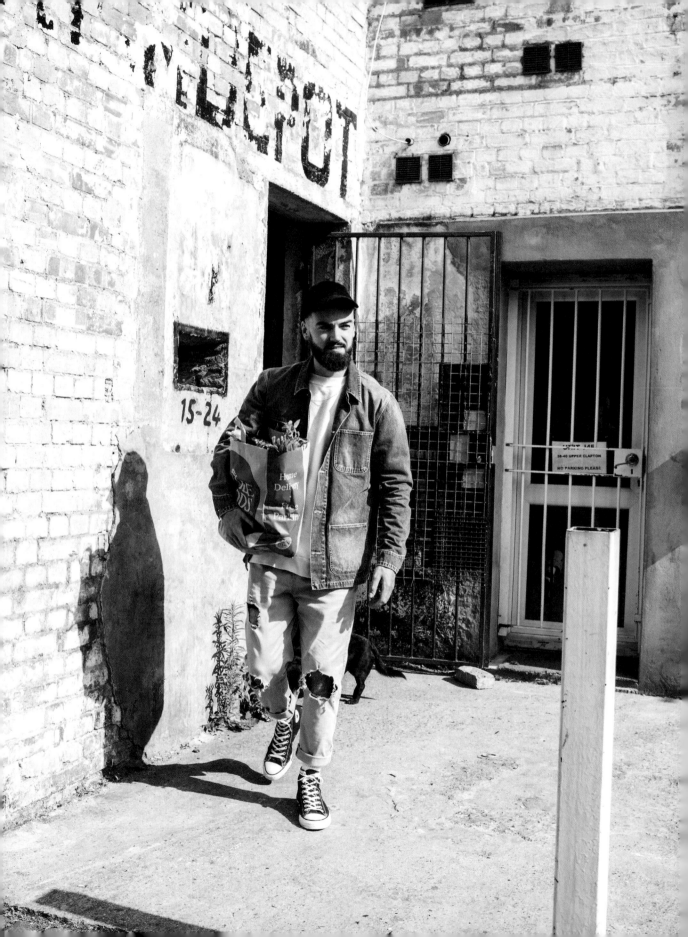

AUBERGINE "BACON"

Here is a soy-free bacon alternative that is so surprising – the aubergine tastes incredible with a smoky flavour and it can get super-crisp. Make sure you either have a mandoline or very sharp knife for slicing the aubergine. I recommend using a mandoline on its thinnest setting; just be very careful and use a hand-guard.

SERVES 5

1 medium aubergine (eggplant)

For the marinade:

2 tbsp maple syrup

2 tbsp coconut aminos
(soy-free soy-style sauce)

2 tbsp soy-free miso

1 tbsp pomegranate molasses

2 tsp smoked paprika

$\frac{1}{4}$ tsp garlic powder

$\frac{1}{2}$ tsp liquid smoke

Preheat the oven to 150°C (300°F) and line a baking tray with greaseproof paper.

First up, mix together all the marinade ingredients in a small mixing bowl.

Top and tail the aubergine and cut it down to a manageable size for your mandoline. Slice into approximately 2-mm ($\frac{1}{16}$-inch) thick slices. Cut each slice in half lengthways. You don't have to do this, it just resembles more of a bacon shape if you do.

Individually coat each piece of aubergine in the marinade, brushing off any excess mixture, then place on the baking tray.

Once you have coated all the aubergine pieces, transfer the tray to the oven and cook for 15 minutes.

Check the aubergine after about 7 minutes and brush on some more of the marinade.

After 15 minutes, remove the tray from the oven. The aubergine should be golden and crisp in places. I like the mixture of crispy ends and soft almost chewy centre.

MAPLE "PUMPKIN PIE" PANCAKES

With their rich sweetness and starchiness, pumpkins and squashes are great in cakes and often found in desserts. They work so well as the main ingredient in these breakfast pancakes and this recipe couldn't be simpler. I usually roast a pumpkin or squash the day before if I know I'm making these for breakfast as the mix works better when the pumpkin is cold.

MAKES 8–10 PANCAKES

1 medium-sized pumpkin or squash (e.g. butternut squash or sugar pumpkin)

180g (2 cups) porridge oats

280ml (1$\frac{1}{4}$ cups) almond Milk (see page 12)

4 tbsp maple syrup

pinch sea salt

1 tsp baking powder

squeeze of lemon juice

1 tbsp coconut oil, for frying

To serve:

3 tbsp coconut yogurt

50ml (3$\frac{1}{2}$ tbsp) maple syrup

handful of walnuts

handful of pumpkin seeds

handful of fruit, such as physalis

The day before, preheat the oven to 180°C (350°F). Roast the pumpkin or squash whole on a tray in the oven for an hour or so, until soft. Set aside until the next day.

The next day, scoop out the flesh and discard the seeds and skin. You will need 120g ($\frac{3}{4}$ cup) for this recipe.

When you're ready to make the pancakes, tip the oats into a blender and blitz on full speed for around 30 seconds. You should be left with a super-fine flour like oat powder.

Add the rest of the ingredients to the blender and pulse it a few times then open and mix with a spatula. Blend again, for about 30 seconds, or until you can see that everything has mixed together well.

Preheat a non-stick pan over a very low heat and lightly grease with the coconut oil. The pan is hot enough when a tiny bit of batter dropped in sizzles. When it is ready, pour the batter directly from the blender jug or ladle it in. I usually make 7.5-cm (3-inch) pancakes which is around 5 tbsp batter.

Cook each pancake for 2–3 minutes on each side. Carefully grease the pan with coconut oil between each pancake to stop them from sticking. I use kitchen paper to rub the oil into the pan.

Once you've cooked all the pancakes, stack them up and serve with coconut yogurt, a drizzle of maple syrup, and a sprinkle of walnuts, pumpkin seeds and fruit.

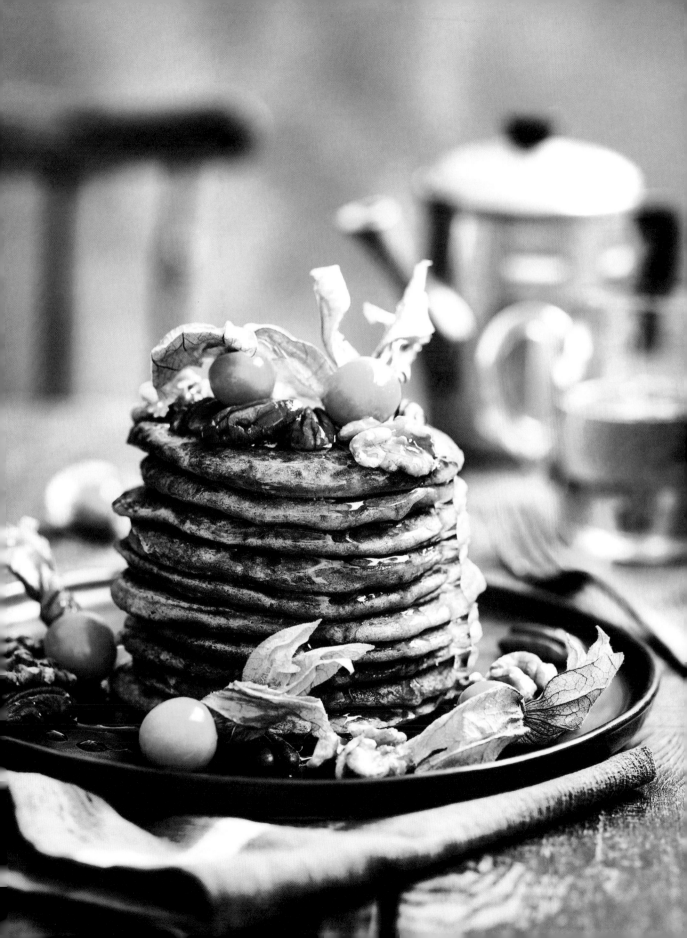

TROPICAL
CHIA SEED PUDDING

Chia seeds are another superfood that I love to work into my breakfasts. They are an excellent source of vital omega-3 fatty acids. Here, I have given them a tropical twist.

SERVES 2–3

5 tbsp chia seeds

240ml (1 cup) filtered cold water

1 frozen banana

1 ripe mango, peeled and cubed

250ml (1 cup) coconut milk

1 tsp vanilla extract

1/2 tsp fresh turmeric (optional)

Toppings:

1 passion fruit, pulp scooped out

2 tbsp coconut flakes

2 tbsp coconut yogurt

small handful of fresh mint, chopped

zest of 1 lime

mango slices

First up, we need to transform the chia seeds. Mix them in a bowl with the water, then pop the bowl in the fridge to let the chia seeds soak for at least 30 minutes. I soak mine overnight.

Meanwhile prepare the other ingredients. Add the banana, half of the chopped mango, the coconut milk, vanilla extract and turmeric to a blender and blitz for 30 seconds, or until smooth.

Blend the rest of the mango into a puree. I keep this to drizzle over the top of the pudding.

Add the banana and mango mix to the soaked chia seeds, mix well and spoon into breakfast bowls.

Top with beautiful passion fruit, coconut flakes and yogurt, fresh mint, lime zest, pureed mango and slices of mango.

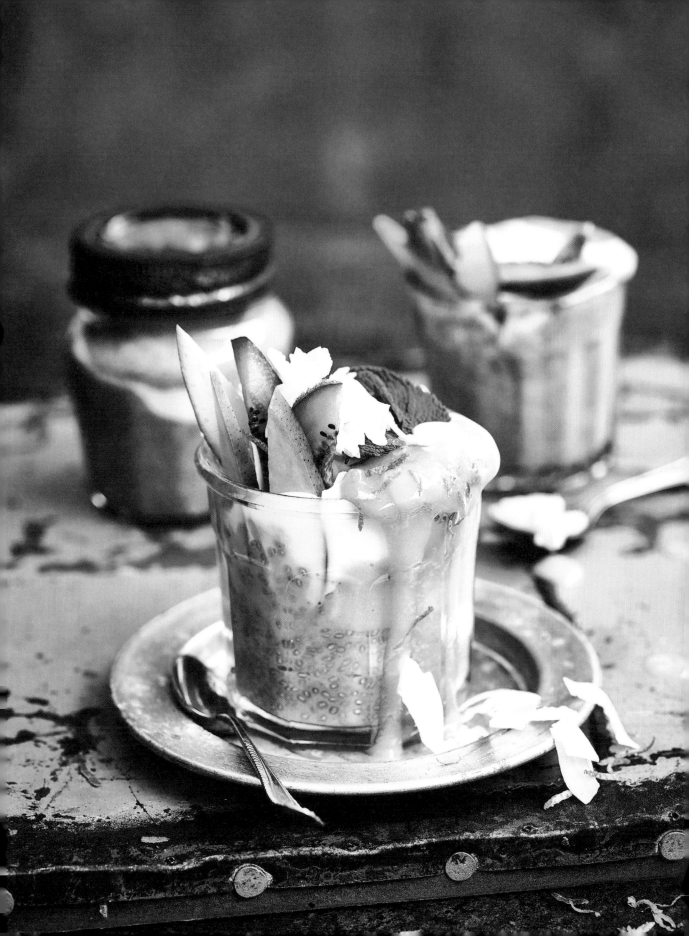

FRUITY QUINOA SALAD

Quinoa is literally a superfood; it's one of the most protein-rich foods we can eat. I jazz it up in this breakfast dish – it works so well with nuts and fruit and is great for a pre-made, on-the-go breakfast. This combination works so well for me but adapt the salad to your taste.

SERVES 2–3

200g (1 cup) quinoa, cooked and chilled

5 tbsp agave nectar

zest and juice of 1 lime

2 tbsp finely chopped fresh mint

2 tbsp coconut flakes

1 tbsp chia seeds

Topping suggestions:

handful of blueberries

handful of strawberries

1 kiwi, peeled and sliced

1 apple, peeled, cored and chopped

1 passion fruit, pulp scooped out

handful of raspberries

handful of cherries

3 tbsp pistachios, shelled

Add the cooked quinoa to a mixing bowl, then stir in the agave nectar, lime zest and juice, mint, coconut and chia seeds. Stir well so that the quinoa is well coated in the sweet, limey goodness.

Spoon into breakfast bowls and top with beautiful fresh fruit and pistachio nuts.

You could also top the salad with coconut yogurt. Simple!

GAZ'S GRANOLA WITH CARAMELIZED CHERRIES

My granola couldn't be simpler. Feel free to use this recipe just as a guide and choose the combination of nuts and seeds you prefer. I highly recommend the caramelized cherries with it, though.

MAKES APPROXIMATELY 5 SERVINGS

180g (2 cups) old-fashioned rolled oats

30g (¼ cup) raw walnut pieces

30g (¼ cup) flaked almonds

30g (¼ cup) coconut flakes

30g (¼ cup) seeds (pumpkin, linseeds, sesame, sunflower, chia, hemp)

60g (½ cup) dried fruit (apricot, raisins, mango, cherries)

1 tbsp coconut oil, melted

2 tbsp maple syrup or agave nectar

For the caramelized cherries:

200g (2 cups) cherries

1 tsp coconut oil

1 tbsp coconut sugar

Preheat the oven to 180°C (350°F).

Throw the oats, nuts, coconut flakes, seeds, dried fruit, coconut oil and maple syrup or agave nectar into a big bowl and mix. Make sure everything gets a good coating of coconut oil and syrup. Be flexible – if you need more of either syrup or oil, just add it.

Line a baking tray with greaseproof paper. Spread the granola mixture out evenly over the tray. Place in the oven to bake for 8–10 minutes, stirring halfway through cooking. (The outside bits will cook quicker.)

Once golden, remove from the oven. The smell will be unbelievable. Leave to cool, then transfer to a storage jar (it will keep fresh for at least a week) or add a serving to your breakfast bowl.

To make the cherries, simply remove the stalks then cut around the stone. Twist the side away from the stone, then remove the stone from the other half. Once you've halved and de-stoned all the cherries, preheat a non-stick saucepan over a medium heat.

Add the coconut oil, followed by the cherries. Sauté for 2 minutes, stirring often, before adding the coconut sugar. Turn the heat down low and cook for a further 2 minutes, stirring often.

Remove from the heat and spoon those juicy, caramelized cherries over the top of the granola. Serve with a big spoonful of dairy-free yogurt and fresh mint, if liked.

MOROCCAN CHICKPEA "OMELETTE"

Witness the magic of chickpeas... This dish resembles an omelette and, if I can say so myself, tastes even better. I have thrown in some North African flavours to give it a Moroccan twist.

MAKES 1 LARGE "OMELETTE"

For the "omelette":

120g (1 cup) chickpea (gram) flour

1 tsp ras el hanout

$\frac{1}{2}$ tsp ground cumin

$\frac{1}{4}$ tsp cayenne pepper

$\frac{1}{4}$ tsp paprika

$\frac{1}{4}$ tsp ground turmeric

$\frac{1}{4}$ tsp chopped fresh thyme

pinch sea salt and cracked black pepper

2 tbsp nutritional yeast

1 tsp baking powder

approximately 250ml (1 cup) water

Filling:

1 red (bell) pepper

1 small red onion

6 cherry tomatoes

10 pitted green olives

handful of spinach

a little olive oil, for frying

Toppings:

handful of fresh baby spinach

1 tbsp of a hummus from page 87

sliced avocado

First up, you will need a large mixing bowl. Add all the omelette ingredients to the bowl apart from the water. Give it a thorough mix, then whisk in enough water until you have a pancake batter consistency.

Cover the batter and pop it in the fridge for 15 minutes while you prepare your filling ingredients.

Finely slice the red pepper and red onion. Thin, even slices work best for this dish. Simply halve the tomatoes and chop the olives into 3. Make sure the spinach has been washed.

Preheat a large, non-stick, oven-proof frying pan and add a small drop of olive oil. (I use a 28-cm [11-inch] pan.) Preheat your grill (broiler).

Add the peppers and red onion and sauté over a medium heat for 2 minutes, stirring often. Once the peppers and onion are soft, remove them from the pan and add them to a bowl with the tomatoes, olives and spinach.

Turn the heat down low and add a touch more oil if you think it needs it. Ladle in the batter, then quickly follow with a good covering of the pepper and spinach mix.

Cook on a low heat for 3 minutes before placing the pan under your grill just to cook the top. Cook for around 3–4 minutes or until golden.

Slide the omelette onto a warm plate and top with lightly dressed spinach, hummus and avocado.

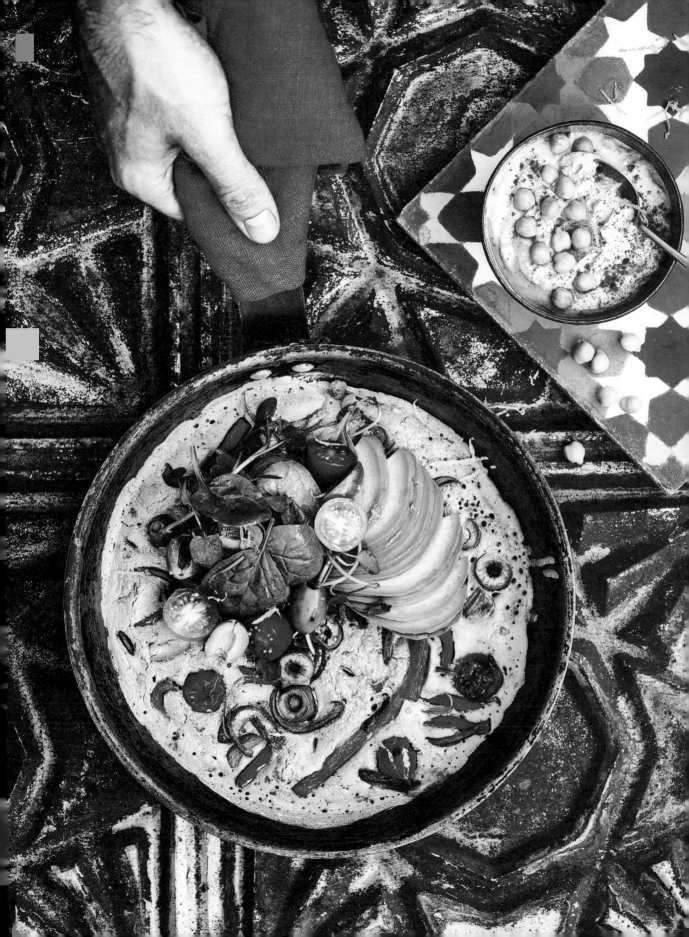

SOUPS

Gaz's Super
Green Gazpacho

Pea Velouté with
Beetroot Ravioli

Peppery Purple Soup

Fragrant Parsnip
& Lentil Soup

Sweet & Spicy Broth

Bountiful Roasted
Butternut Soup, Crispy
Sage & Smoky Seeds

GAZ'S SUPER GREEN GAZPACHO

So vibrant, bold, refreshing and peppery, this is one of the simplest summer soups to make but it's important to season it properly. Keep checking the taste until it's powerful. The rose-petal ice cubes will take your gazpacho to the next level and really impress your guests. They are the simplest things to make but they just look so beautiful and they add a great floral note. The gazpacho is best served straight-out-of-the-fridge cold, so make it at least an hour before serving.

SERVES 4–5

4 handfuls of spinach, washed

3 garlic cloves

1 cucumber, deseeded and chopped

½ green chilli, deseeded

handful of fresh mint

handful of fresh parsley

handful of fresh basil

1 over-ripe avocado, peeled and de-stoned

5 spring onions (scallions)

5 tbsp coconut yogurt

2 tbsp extra virgin olive oil

2 tbsp white wine vinegar

approximately 1 litre (4 cups) filtered water

pinch salt and pepper

a little lemon juice, optional

To serve:

dried rose petals

cherry tomatoes

sugar snap peas

watercress

avocado roses (see opposite)

First up, ahead of making the soup, make the spectacular rose-petal ice cubes. Fill an ice-cube tray up with water and drop 3–4 rose petals into each cube. Place in the freezer to freeze solid.

Put all the soup ingredients, except the water and seasoning, in a blender – you will more than likely have to do this in stages as not everything will fit into the blender in its solid form. Once everything is in the blender and half blended, pour the water in. Keep adding the water and blending until you've reached a smooth, soupy consistency.

The key with gazpacho is to make sure the soup is super-smooth. There should be no bits, so if your blender isn't very powerful and doesn't completely blend the soup, just pass it through a sieve.

Pour into a container and check the seasoning. This is really crucial: be generous with the salt and pepper as you want to really bring out the flavours. Add lemon juice instead of additional salt if you prefer. This will also make the flavours pop.

Chill the soup in the fridge until you're ready to serve; it's as easy as that!

To serve, pour the soup into your serving bowls. Top with 3 rose-petal ice cubes per person, a few cherry tomatoes and sugar snap peas, some watercress and an avocado rose (if you really want to wow your guests). To find out how to make an avocado rose, check out my first ever YouTube video (when I was kind of shy!).

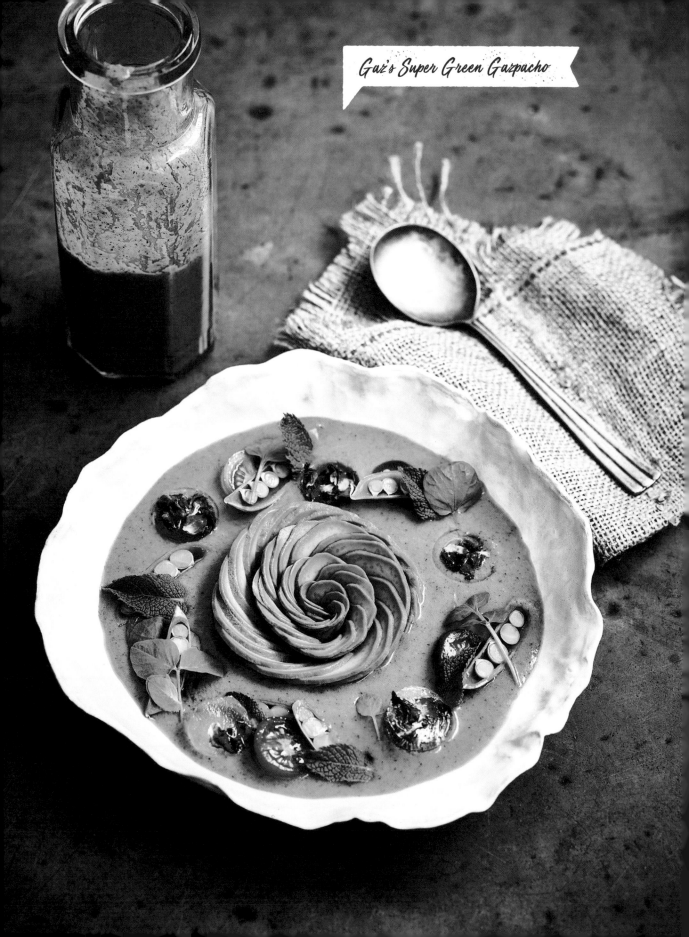

Gaz's Super Green Gazpacho

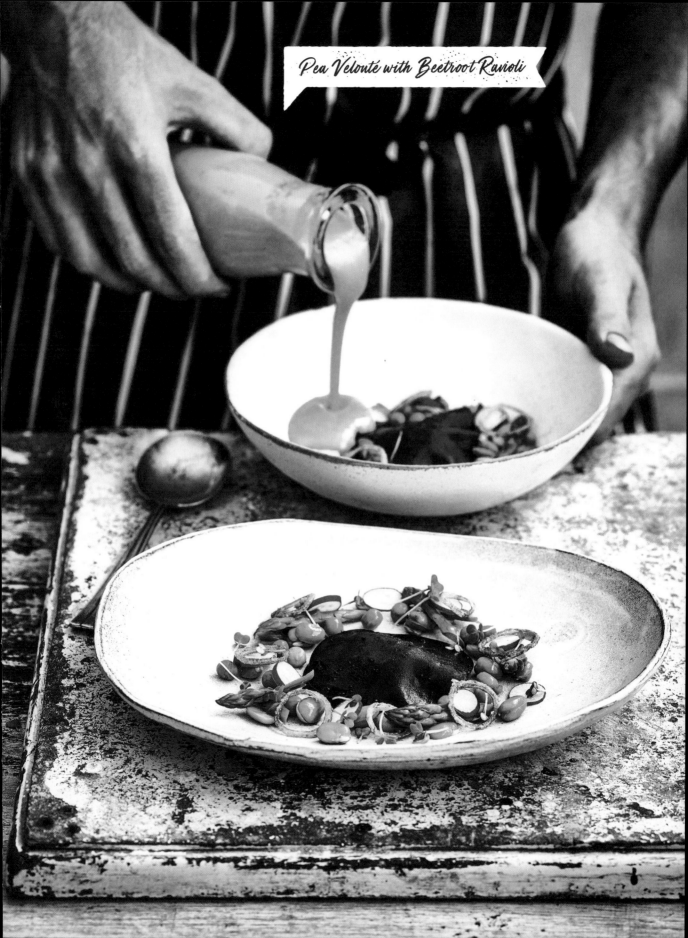

Pea Velouté with Beetroot Ravioli

PEA VELOUTÉ WITH BEETROOT RAVIOLI

I came up with this recipe when I was working at Le Gallois restaurant; it was a huge hit throughout spring and summer. Beautiful peas, wasabi and beetroot are an incredible combination. The soup was served in a jug next to a bowl filled with the raw beetroot ravioli, spring greens and crispy shallot rings. The pea velouté is really quick and simple to make and is just as tasty on its own, but I definitely recommend serving it with the ravioli and garnishes for a special occasion.

SERVES 2

For the velouté:

2 tbsp extra virgin olive oil

5 shallots, finely chopped

pinch salt and pepper

900g (approximately 7 cups) frozen peas

750ml (3 cups) Vegetable Stock (see page 31)

470ml (2 cups) almond Milk (see page 12)

juice of $\frac{1}{2}$ lemon

For the beetroot ravioli:

1 beetroot (beet), peeled

1 tbsp white wine vinegar

juice of $\frac{1}{2}$ lemon

1 tbsp maple syrup

$\frac{1}{4}$ tsp poppy seeds

$\frac{1}{4}$ tsp sesame seeds

5 tbsp "Cream Cheese" (see page 15)

$\frac{1}{4}$ tsp wasabi paste

For the crispy shallot rings:

1 shallot, peeled and cut into fine rings

60g ($\frac{1}{2}$ cup) gluten-free flour blend

pinch salt and pepper

750ml (3 cups) vegetable oil, for frying

To garnish:

handful of lightly steamed asparagus, broad beans and peas

sliced radishes

cress

First up, make the soup, which can be made ahead of serving and chilled.

In a large saucepan over a low heat, add the olive oil and then chopped shallots with a pinch of seasoning. Sweat the shallots until they are translucent. Keep stirring and be careful not to burn them.

Once the shallots are cooked, add half of the peas, stir in and let them defrost and cook in the pan for around 5 minutes. Stir in the stock and milk then cover the saucepan and bring the soup to a light simmer. Simmer for 4 minutes.

When the soup is lightly simmering, add the remaining peas followed by some more seasoning. (Adding half of the frozen peas later is a little trick to keep the soup super-green in colour and fresh in taste.) Allow to cook for 2 minutes more while you set up your blender.

Remove the soup from the heat, pour into the blender and blitz quickly. You will probably have to do this in batches depending on the size of your blender. Make sure the soup is super-smooth, as if it has any bits it can't be classed as a velouté. To be extra sure, you can pass the soup through a sieve.

Once the soup is blended, stir in the lemon juice for additional seasoning. Then set aside, chill until needed or serve on its own straight away.

To make the beetroot ravioli, slice the beetroot as thinly as possible into rounds using a mandoline on its thinnest setting. Be careful and make sure you use the hand guard. You will need two good-sized beetroot discs per person.

Now mix the vinegar, lemon juice, maple syrup, and poppy and sesame seeds in a bowl, then add the beetroot slices and marinate in this mixture for at least 30 minutes.

Meanwhile, make the filling: simply mix the cream cheese together with the wasabi in a bowl.

After the beetroot has marinated, place 5 slices on a baking tray. (A little tip is to make sure the smaller beetroot discs are on the bottom.) Spoon a teaspoon of the wasabi cream cheese into the centre of each slice, then place another beetroot slice over the top. Do this delicately to keep the shape looking like a ravioli. Pop the ravioli in the fridge to chill until serving.

To make the crispy shallot rings, toss the rings in a mixture of the flour and seasoning. Fill a saucepan no more than half full with the vegetable oil and heat until a piece of bread dropped in sizzles and browns within a few seconds. (If using a fryer, set it to around 170°C [340°F].) Swiftly and carefully, lower the rings into the oil to fry for 1 minute or until golden. Do not drop them in all at once as they will stick together. Remove from the oil and place on kitchen paper to drain off any excess oil. Do this just before serving so they stay crisp.

To serve, place a beetroot ravioli in the centre of a serving bowl. Dot a few steamed vegetables and radish slices around, followed by a few crispy shallot rings. Sprinkle over some peppery cress. Serve the soup in a jug on the side, piping hot, for your guests to pour over.

PEPPERY PURPLE SOUP

This is the deepest purple soup made from red cabbage and red onion. Red cabbage is so nutritious and not many people know how versatile it is – this soup is a great way to celebrate it. The thyme complements the flavour perfectly, and the balsamic and apple add delicious sweetness.

SERVES 5

2 red onions

1 medium red cabbage

1 large sweet apple

2 tbsp extra virgin olive oil

4 sprigs fresh thyme, leaves picked

750ml (3 cups) Vegetable Stock (see page 31)

470ml (2 cups) almond Milk (see page 12)

2 tbsp balsamic vinegar

pinch salt and pepper

To garnish:

slices of apple

spoonful of "Crème Fraîche" (see page 17)

sprinkling of fresh thyme leaves and chopped chives

Peel and slice the onions roughly but just make sure all the pieces are a similar size so they cook evenly. Peel the outer layers of the red cabbage and give it a rinse. Cut it in half, then half again. Shred the cabbage quarters evenly. Grate the apple flesh, avoiding the bitter core.

Preheat a large saucepan over a medium heat and add the olive oil. Once hot, add the onion, cabbage and apple. Follow this with a pinch of seasoning and the thyme. Seasoning early helps build a depth of flavour.

Cook for around 4 minutes, stirring often to avoid anything burning. The mixture should have halved in volume after 4 minutes and it's now time to add the stock, milk and balsamic vinegar. Give everything a good stir, then pop the lid on. Simmer for 10-15 minutes, then check the red cabbage is soft. If so, start to blend. For this type of soup, I am not too bothered about how smooth it is; in fact, it's nice with a bit of texture, so by all means use a hand stick blender as it's a lot easier.

Once blitzed, check one last time for seasoning. I sometimes add an additional sprinkling of cracked black pepper as it works really well with the red cabbage. Serve the punchy peppery purple goodness topped with fresh apple slices, a spoonful of crème fraîche and a sprinkling of thyme and chives.

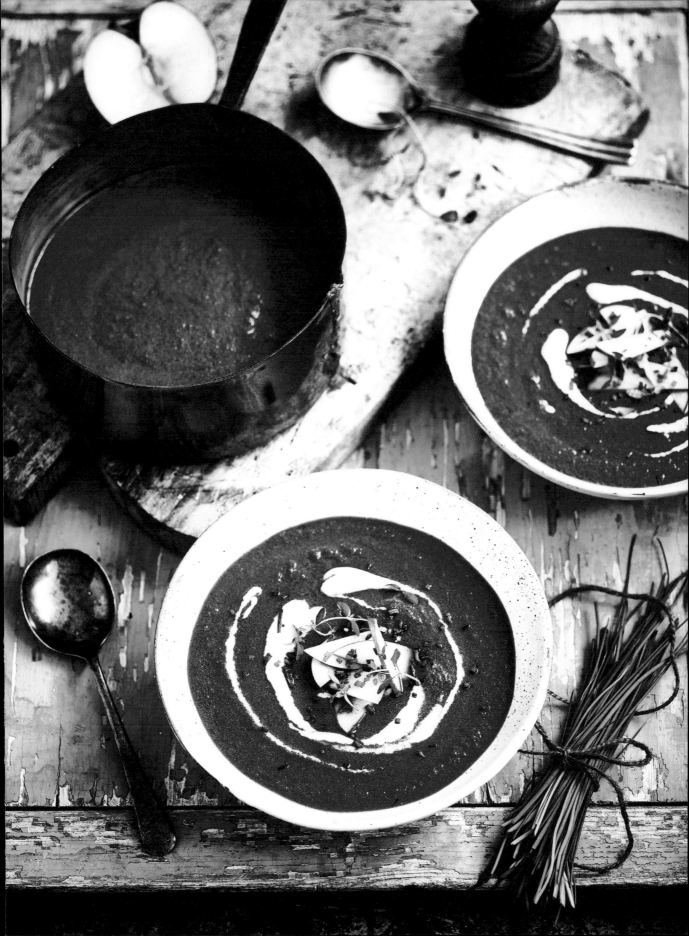

FRAGRANT PARSNIP & LENTIL SOUP

Similar to a dhal, this aromatic soup is rich and creamy, and is perfect on a cold day. Lentils are a great form of fibre and help to lower blood cholesterol. Top with a beautiful spicy carrot and coriander salad and crispy parsnips to make it extra special.

SERVES 4–5

1 tbsp coconut oil

1 medium white onion, finely sliced

1 tsp chopped fresh ginger

2 garlic cloves, crushed

1 tsp ground cumin

1 tsp ground coriander

$\frac{1}{4}$ tsp ground turmeric

$\frac{1}{4}$ tsp chilli powder

$\frac{1}{4}$ tsp ground cardamom

$\frac{1}{4}$ tsp ground cinnamon

5 parsnips, peeled and cubed

200g (1 cup) red lentils, rinsed

720ml (3 cups) Vegetable Stock (see page 31)

480ml (2 cups) soy milk or almond Milk (see page 12)

pinch salt and pepper

sprinkle of black onion seeds, to serve

For the parsnip crisps:

1 parsnip, peeled

3 tbsp vegetable oil

pinch salt and pepper

For the carrot & coriander salad:

1 carrot

1 red onion, finely sliced

handful of fresh coriander (cilantro), chopped

1 green chilli, finely chopped

Preheat the oven to 180°C (350°F).

First make the soup. Heat the coconut oil in a large, lidded saucepan over a medium heat and add the onion, ginger and garlic. Stir for 1 minute, then add all of the spices. Season with salt and pepper. Cook for 2–3 minutes, stirring often. (At this point the smell will be incredible.)

Add the parsnips to the saucepan, then the lentils. Quickly give it all a stir, then pour in the vegetable stock and the milk. The milk helps the parsnips retain their colour. Pop the lid on, turn the heat down to low and simmer for 20 minutes.

Meanwhile, make the parsnip crisps: peel the parsnip flesh into ribbons using a peeler into a bowl.

Pour over the oil, sprinkle with seasoning and give them a good mix, making sure all the ribbons are coated with oil.

Line a baking tray with greaseproof paper, then spread the parsnip ribbons out on the tray. You don't have to be overly neat, just make sure they aren't all on top of one another. Roast the parsnips in the oven on the middle shelf for 10–12 minutes. Once cooked, sprinkle over salt to keep them crisp, then set aside.

Double check the lentils and parsnips in the soup are tender after 20 minutes and remove the saucepan from the heat. Use a hand blender to blend the soup in the pan. It doesn't have to be super-smooth. If your soup is on the thick side, add more water or milk.

Once the soup is blended and just before serving, prepare the carrot salad. Grate the carrot into a bowl, add the onion slices, coriander and chilli. Stir to combine.

Serve the soup topped with the carrot salad, crispy parsnips and a sprinkle of black onion seeds.

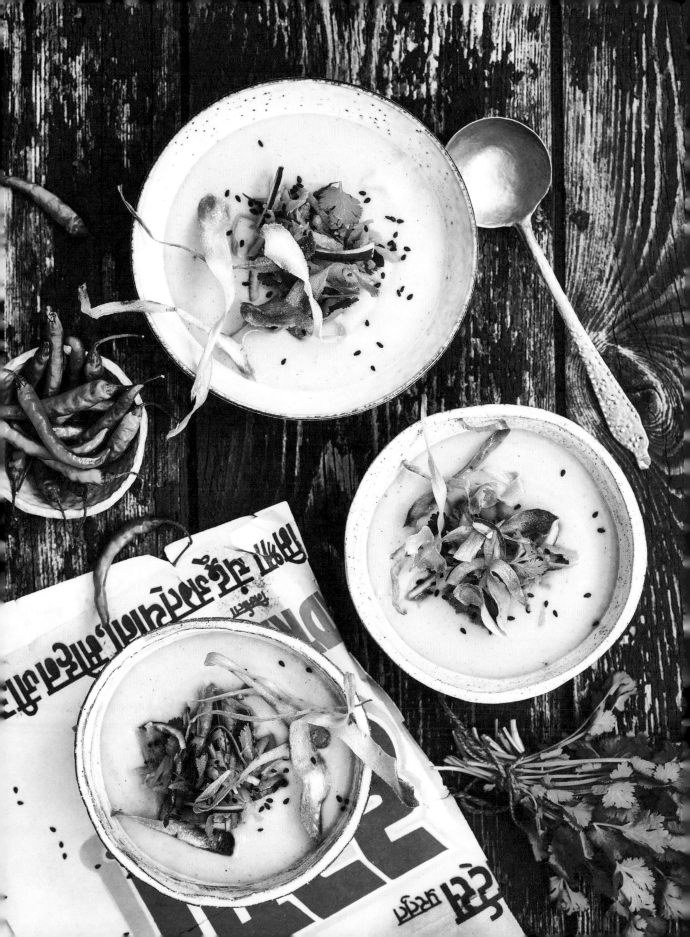

SWEET & SPICY BROTH

Packed full of punchy flavours and made in around 20 minutes, this fiery yet sweet soup is delicious. Add rice noodles if you want to turn it into more of a meal.

SERVES 4

2 tbsp sesame oil

2 tbsp fresh ginger, finely chopped

2 garlic cloves, crushed

1 medium red chilli, deseeded and finely chopped

180g (6^1/$_4$oz) firm tofu, cut into 1-cm (^{3}/$_8$-inch) cubes

70g (1 cup) shiitake mushrooms, sliced

1 litre (4 cups) hot Vegetable Stock (see page 31)

3 tbsp light soy sauce

1 tbsp miso paste

1 tbsp rice wine vinegar

3 tbsp maple syrup

70g (1 cup) fresh or canned bean sprouts

35g (^{1}/$_2$ cup) fresh samphire

100g (1 cup) pak choi leaves

4 spring onions (scallions), thinly sliced diagonally, to serve

1 tbsp black and white sesame seeds, to serve

Preheat a large wok or saucepan over a high heat. Add the sesame oil and wait for the wok to get super-hot. When the oil is almost smoking, throw in the ginger, garlic and chilli. Sauté for 1 minute before adding the tofu and mushrooms.

Toss and stir the mixture while cooking for a further 2 minutes, then leave to cook for around 30 seconds more.

Turn the heat down low and add the vegetable stock, soy sauce, miso, vinegar and maple syrup. Let the soup simmer away for 5 minutes, then add the bean sprouts and samphire. Cook for 2 more minutes. Add the pak choi, let it wilt, then remove the wok from the heat.

Serve the soup straight away, topped with the spring onions and a sprinkle of mixed sesame seeds.

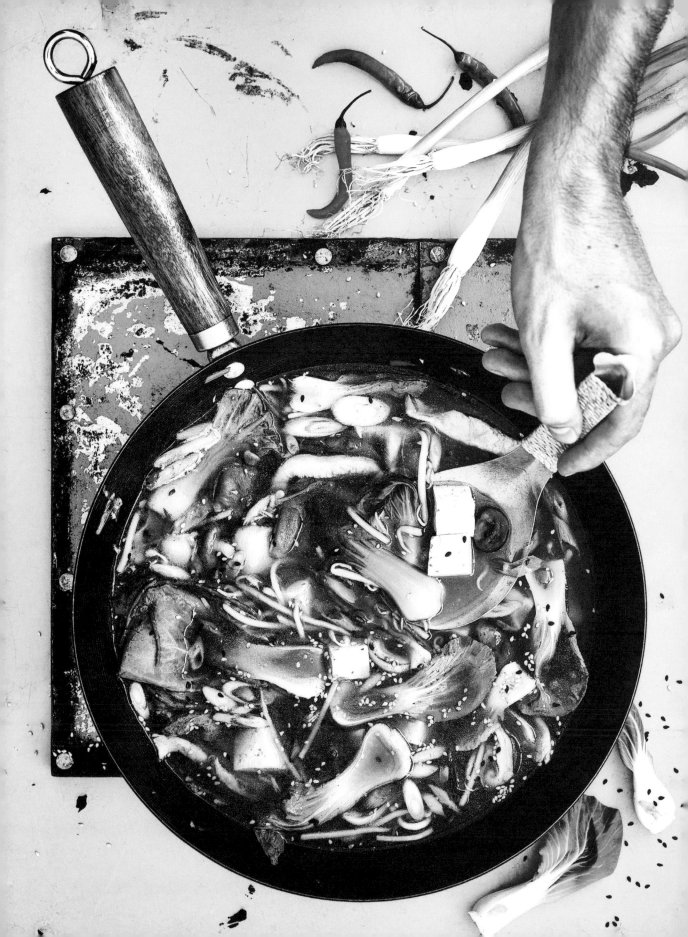

BOUNTIFUL ROASTED BUTTERNUT SOUP, CRISPY SAGE & SMOKY SEEDS

If I had to choose between all the soups in my book, this one would be my number one. Butternut squash is my favourite vegetable and here the spices, coconut and sage magnify its incredible flavour. Rather than wasting the nutritious squash seeds, this recipe makes good use of them.

SERVES 4

For the soup:

1 large butternut squash

4 garlic cloves, peeled

3 tbsp coconut oil, melted

1 tsp cayenne pepper

1 tsp dried oregano

1 tsp dried sage

1 tsp fresh thyme leaves

1 tsp smoked paprika

1 tsp dried chilli flakes

pinch sea salt and pepper

1 large white onion, finely chopped

1 x 400-ml (14-oz) can coconut milk

480ml (2 cups) Vegetable Stock (see page 31)

For the smoky seeds:

seeds from the butternut squash

2 tbsp maple syrup

1 tbsp coconut oil, melted

1 tsp smoked paprika

pinch sea salt

For the crispy sage leaves:

2–3 tbsp extra virgin olive oil

handful of fresh sage leaves

To serve:

dairy-free soy cream (optional)

sprinkle of dried chilli flakes (optional)

Preheat the oven to 180°C (350°F).

First up, cut the squash in half down the middle, scoop out the seeds and set them aside. Cut each half into half again lengthways. I recommend using a serrated knife for cutting squash as the skin is quite tough.

Place the squash and garlic cloves in a roasting tray, drizzle over 2 tablespoons of the coconut oil and sprinkle over all of the herbs and spices. Get your hands involved and make sure the squash quarters are well coated in the herbs and spices.

Pop the squash in the oven to roast for 45 minutes to 1 hour, or until soft.

Meanwhile, grab the squash seeds. Wash them in a colander and get rid of the stringy bits, so you're left with clean, shiny seeds. Pat them dry and add them to a bowl with the maple syrup, coconut oil, smoked paprika and salt. Give the seeds a mix to make sure they are all coated.

Line a baking tray with greaseproof paper and spread the seeds out evenly. Roast on the bottom shelf of the oven for around 20 minutes until golden.

Once the butternut squash is cooked, remove from the oven and set aside.

Preheat a large saucepan over a low heat with the remaining coconut oil, the chopped onion and a sprinkling of seasoning. Sweat the onion for 2–3 minutes, or until soft.

Meanwhile, scoop the squash flesh from the skins using a large spoon, then add it to the saucepan, along with the roasted garlic cloves. Pour in the coconut milk and the vegetable stock. Put the lid on and simmer the soup for 5 minutes to let the flavours get to know each other.

While the soup is simmering, preheat a small, non-stick frying pan over a medium heat with the olive oil. Once hot, add the sage leaves and let them cook for 30 seconds on each side. Remove from the pan and transfer to kitchen paper to soak up any excess oil. Sprinkle with salt to keep them crisp.

Blitz the soup in a blender or with a hand stick blender. I like my squash soup super-smooth so I use a powerful blender. Bowl up the soup and serve with the crispy sage, smoky seeds, a swirl of soy cream and sprinkle of dried chilli flakes, if liked.

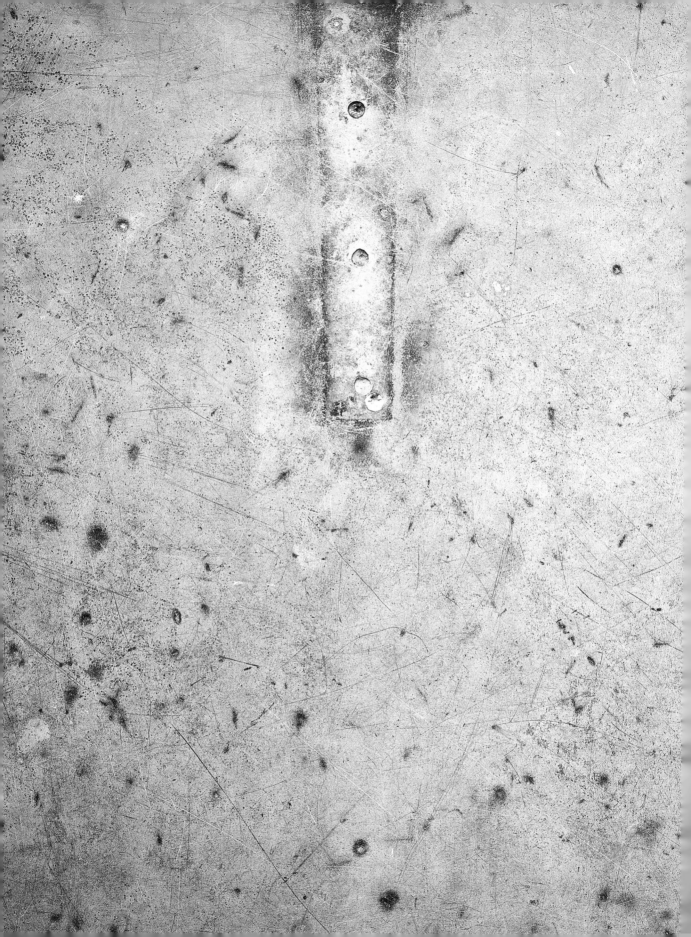

SNACKS & BITES

Spinach & Basil
Buckwheat Crêpes

Loaded Nachos with
Spicy Black Beans, Nacho
"Cheese" Sauce & Salsa

Potato & Leek Croquettes
with Relish

Raw Spaghetti with
Avocado & Chilli Sauce &
Almond "Parmesan" Crumb

Tofu Tikka Kebabs
with Carrot Salad

Carrot & Red Onion Bhajis
with Mint Yogurt

Gaz's "Guac"

Super Pink Beetroot Hummus

Pumpkin & Sage Hummus

Paprika & Thyme Hummus

Peri Peri Falafel with
Tahini Dressing

Roasted Balsamic Beetroot
& Shallot Tarts

Ultimate Vegan Baguettes

Spicy Sweetcorn & Kale Potato
Rösti with Mango Salsa

Summer Rolls with
Sweet Chilli Dip

Kentucky Fried Chick'n

SPINACH & BASIL BUCKWHEAT CRÊPES

**These speedy, nutrient-rich crêpes are the perfect light lunch.
Fill them with a savoury filling of your choice.**

MAKES 7–8 CRÊPES

360ml (1½ cups) almond
Milk (see page 12)

2 handfuls of spinach
leaves, washed

handful of fresh basil leaves

180g (1½ cups) buckwheat flour

pinch sea salt and pepper

juice of ½ lemon

1 tbsp coconut oil, for frying

2 tbsp Pepper & Tomato
Relish (see page 80)

Filling suggestions:

Meltable "Mozzarella"
(see page 18)

steamed asparagus

red onion, sliced

fresh basil, torn

Blitz the milk in a blender with the spinach and basil until it's smooth and super-green.

Add the flour to a mixing bowl and whisk in enough of the green milk mix to turn it into a smooth light batter. Season with salt and pepper and stir in the lemon juice.

Pop the batter in the fridge to settle for 10 minutes while you prepare your fillings.

Preheat a large, non-stick frying pan (or, even better, a crêpe pan) over a low heat. Rub with some coconut oil before it gets hot.

When the pan is hot, ladle in enough batter to cover the pan, swirling the batter around to help spread it thinly and evenly. Cook for 1–2 minutes on each side, or until golden.

Continue until you have cooked all the crêpes, then serve with your chosen fillings and the Pepper & Tomato Relish.

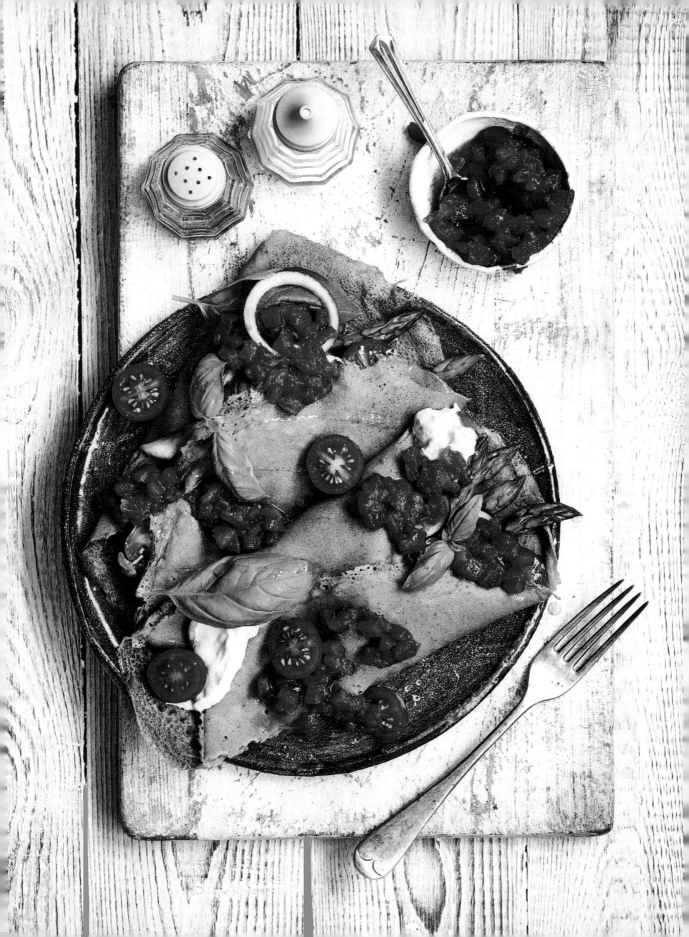

LOADED NACHOS WITH SPICY BLACK BEANS, NACHO "CHEESE" SAUCE & SALSA

Sometimes at the weekend I crave a great stack of these nachos. I've made sure there are loads of nutrients in this dish, which makes them an even bigger treat.

SERVES 4

For the crispy baked nachos:

5 tortillas, cut into triangles

2 tbsp vegetable oil

For the nacho "cheese" sauce:

75g (½ cup) raw cashew nuts, soaked in boiling water for 10 minutes

180ml (¾ cup) almond Milk (see page 12)

2 tbsp fresh lemon juice

2 tbsp nutritional yeast

¼ tsp mustard powder

¼ tsp dried chilli flakes

pinch garlic powder

For the red pepper & tomato salsa:

1 red (bell) pepper

handful of cherry tomatoes

1 small red onion, finely chopped

handful of fresh coriander (cilantro), finely chopped

juice of 1 lime

pinch salt and pepper

For the spicy black beans:

1 tbsp coconut oil

1 x 400-g (14-oz) can black beans, drained and rinsed

¼ tsp dried oregano

¼ tsp cayenne pepper

¼ tsp onion powder

¼ tsp paprika

1 tsp Tabasco sauce

Toppings:

avocado

pickled jalapeños

fresh coriander

Preheat the oven to 180°C (350°F) and line a couple of baking trays with greaseproof paper.

Add the tortilla triangles to a mixing bowl, pour over the oil and give them a mix, making sure they are all coated. Spread the tortilla triangles over the prepared baking trays and bake for 10–12 minutes, or until golden and crisp.

To make the nacho cheese sauce, drain the soaked cashews and add to a blender with the rest of the ingredients. Blend until smooth. Cover with cling film (plastic wrap) then place in the fridge until ready to serve.

For the salsa, hold the red pepper directly over the flame of a gas hob to char the skin, turning it around using tongs until it's completely charred. Put the pepper in a bowl quickly and cover with cling film. If you don't have a gas hob, grill (broil) or roast the pepper (see page 80).

Meanwhile, prepare the rest of the salsa ingredients: quarter the cherry tomatoes and add to a bowl with the red onion, fresh coriander and lime juice.

Remove the cling film from the pepper bowl. Cut the pepper into 4 and remove the seeds and stalk. Then, using the back of a small knife, scrape away the charred skin from the flesh. Cube the peeled pepper flesh, then add it to the salsa bowl. Mix well and season, then set aside until you're ready to serve.

Next up, the black beans: melt the coconut oil in a small saucepan, then add the beans with all the herbs and spices, and the Tabasco. Stir over a low heat until piping hot.

To serve, fill a serving bowl with the crispy baked nachos, then the black beans, followed by the salsa. Finally, drizzle the cheesy nacho sauce all over and top with fresh avocado, pickled jalapeños and fresh coriander.

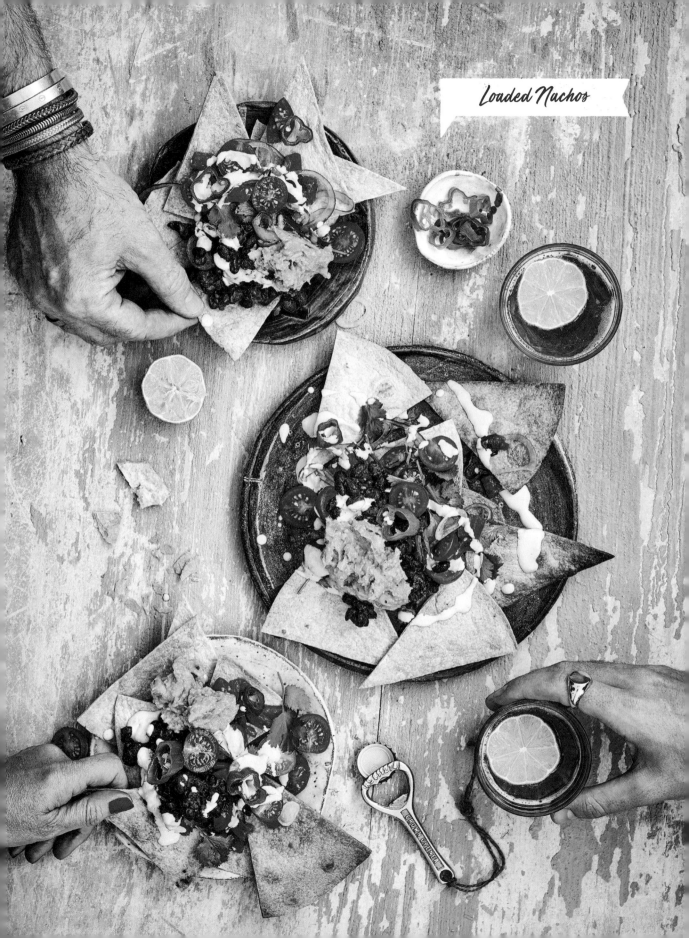

Loaded Nachos

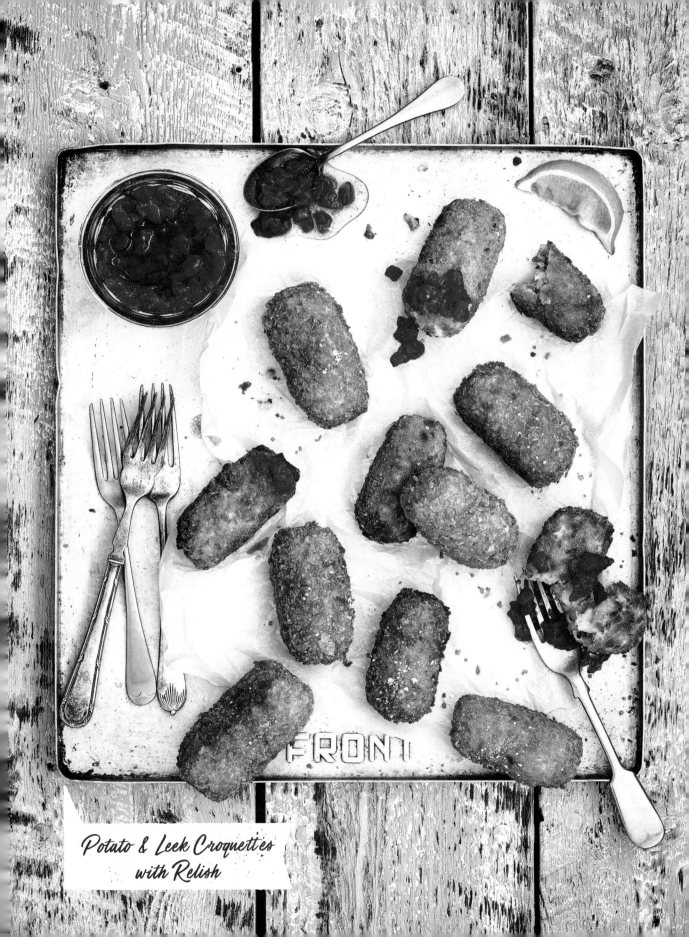

Potato & Leek Croquettes
with Relish

POTATO & LEEK CROQUETTES WITH RELISH

These little heavenly potato pillows are a treat that get me excited every time I think of them. The relish also works with many other dishes and will keep for a few weeks in the fridge. These two go very well together. You can bake the croquettes or fry them in a deep-fat fryer.

MAKES ABOUT 15

For the pepper & tomato relish:

3 red (bell) peppers

7 ripe tomatoes

4 shallots, finely chopped

4 tbsp unrefined caster (granulated) sugar

120ml (½ cup) white wine vinegar

pinch salt and pepper

For the croquettes:

1 large leek

3 tbsp olive oil

3 large Maris Piper potatoes, baked

2 tbsp chives, finely chopped

1 tbsp "Butter" Spread (see page 14)

salt and pepper to taste

50g (1 cup) panko breadcrumbs (or gluten-free breadcrumbs)

5 tbsp cornflour (cornstarch)

60g (½ cup) plain (all-purpose) flour (or gluten-free flour)

1 litre (4 cups) vegetable oil, if frying

Preheat the oven to 180°C (350°F) and start making the relish. Place the peppers on a baking tray and bake in the preheated oven for 30 minutes, until they are slightly charred. Alternatively, hold each pepper directly over the flame of a gas hob to char the skin, turning it around using tongs until it's completely charred. Either way, put the peppers in a bowl and cover with cling film (plastic wrap).

Fill a small bowl with boiling water and another with ice-cold water. Lightly score a cross on the bottom of each tomato, plunge them into the hot water for 1 minute, then straight into cold water. Peel the skins off and discard.

Once the peppers are cool, deseed them and, using the back of your knife, peel/scrape off the charred skin and discard.

Chop the tomato and pepper flesh into evenly sized pieces. Tip into a heavy-based saucepan with the remaining ingredients. Cook over a very low heat with the lid on, stirring occasionally, for around 40 minutes, or until it's thickened. Remove from the heat and pour into a sterilized 227-g (8-oz) jar or container.

To make the croquettes, peel the top layer off the leek and top and tail it. Rinse under cold water to remove any dirt, then slice into fine rings. Preheat a non-stick frying pan. Add a little olive oil and sauté the leek until soft and slightly golden, then remove from the pan.

Peel the skin off the baked potatoes, then mash. Add to a bowl with the cooked leek, chives, butter and seasoning. Combine everything together and check it's seasoned well. Cover the bowl and place in the fridge.

To cook the croquettes, preheat the oven again to 180°C (350°F) or set up your fryer with vegetable oil to 180°C (350°F). Line a baking tray with greaseproof paper.

In 3 shallow bowls, place the breadcrumbs in one; the cornflour mixed with 5 tablespoons water in another; and the flour in the third. Remove the potato mix from the fridge and mould into even-sized croquette shapes with your hands. Dip each one into the 3 bowls in the following order: flour, wet cornflour mixture, then crumbs.

Place the coated croquettes on the lined baking tray, drizzle over about 2 tbsp olive oil, then bake for 20 minutes, or until golden. If using a fryer, fry for about 4 minutes. Serve hot with the relish.

RAW SPAGHETTI WITH AVOCADO & CHILLI SAUCE & ALMOND "PARMESAN" CRUMB

Fresh, vibrant, filling and nutritious... Oh, and also delectable. This is my go-to, quick raw meal. Omit the nutritional yeast if you'd prefer the dish to be 100% raw. You will need a spiralizer for this recipe.

SERVES 4

1 courgette (zucchini), spiralized

2 carrots, shredded or spiralized

For the avocado & chilli sauce:

1 over-ripe avocado

juice of $\frac{1}{2}$ lemon

3 tbsp avocado oil

1 small garlic clove

handful of fresh basil leaves

3 tbsp raw pine nuts

$\frac{1}{4}$ tsp onion powder

$\frac{1}{2}$ tsp dried chilli flakes

60ml ($\frac{1}{4}$ cup) filtered water

For the almond "parmesan" crumb:

50g ($\frac{1}{2}$ cup) blanched almonds

1 tbsp nutritional yeast

$\frac{1}{2}$ tsp garlic powder

$\frac{1}{4}$ tsp sea salt

To serve:

a few cherry tomatoes

handful of fresh basil leaves

To make the avocado & chilli sauce, simply add all the ingredients to a blender and blitz until smooth. Cover with cling film (plastic wrap) and place in the fridge until ready to serve.

For the almond parmesan crumb, again blitz all the ingredients together in a blender until you have a fine crumb.

To serve, put the spiralized courgette and carrots in a mixing bowl. Spoon in the sauce and give it a good mix to coat the vegetables. Dish up into serving bowls then top with cherry tomatoes, fresh basil and a sprinkle of parmesan crumb.

TOFU TIKKA KEBABS WITH CARROT SALAD

This recipe is great for your friends who say they hate tofu – the flavours are tantalizing. Feel free to add a little extra chilli if you like more of a kick!

MAKES 12 KEBABS

1 x 400-g (14-oz) block of firm tofu, cut into 2-cm (³/₄-inch) cubes

1 red (bell) pepper, cut into 2-cm (³/₄-inch) cubes

1 yellow (bell) pepper, cut into 2-cm (³/₄-inch) cubes

1 large red onion, cut into 2-cm (³/₄-inch) cubes

For the marinade:

250ml (1 cup) plain dairy-free yogurt

2 garlic cloves, crushed

1 tbsp fresh ginger, finely chopped

2 green chillies, finely chopped

1 tbsp ground cumin

1 tbsp ground coriander

2 tbsp fresh lemon juice

1 tsp ground turmeric

1 tsp salt

handful of fresh coriander (cilantro), finely chopped

For the carrot salad:

2 carrots, peeled and grated

1 red onion, finely sliced

handful of fresh coriander (cilantro), finely chopped

1 green chilli, finely sliced

2 tbsp black onion seeds

pinch sea salt

juice of 1 lime

Mix together the marinade ingredients in a large bowl. Add the tofu cubes, pepper and red onion and stir to make sure everything is coated. Cover the bowl and place in the fridge to marinate for at least 1 hour.

Meanwhile, mix together all the salad ingredients and set aside.

If you're using wooden skewers to cook the kebabs, soak them in water to stop them burning in the oven.

Before building your skewers, preheat your oven to 200°C (400°F) and line a baking tray with greaseproof paper.

Start off by threading a piece of pepper on to each skewer; this will stop anything falling off. Follow by a mixture of the rest of the pieces.

Lay the finished skewers on the baking tray, and spoon over any excess marinade. Bake for 25–30 minutes. Eat straight away with the salad.

CARROT & RED ONION BHAJIS WITH MINT YOGURT

These little aromatic crispy balls of goodness are a flavour punch! I like to add a little heat to my bhajis so I recommend serving these with the cooling mint yogurt.

MAKES ABOUT 12

For the bhajis:

2 large red onions, finely sliced

2 carrots, grated

1 tsp sea salt

1 garlic clove, crushed

1 tsp ground turmeric

1 green chilli, finely chopped

handful of fresh coriander (cilantro), roughly chopped

3–4 tbsp chickpea (gram) flour

1–2 tbsp water

1 litre (4 cups) vegetable oil, if frying

For the mint yogurt:

250g (1 cup) coconut yogurt

10-cm (4-inch) piece of cucumber, deseeded and cut into small cubes

handful of fresh mint, finely shredded

juice of $\frac{1}{2}$ lemon

1 garlic clove, crushed

$\frac{1}{2}$ tsp ground cumin

$\frac{1}{2}$ tsp mild chilli powder

Preheat the oven to 200°C (400°F) or set your fryer to heat the vegetable oil to 180°C (350°F) if you prefer to fry your bhajis.

Mix the onions and carrots in a bowl, sprinkle over the salt and stir to combine. Set the bowl aside for 5 minutes. (The salt just breaks down the onions slightly.)

Meanwhile, in a separate bowl, mix all of the yogurt ingredients together, cover with cling film (plastic wrap) and pop in the fridge until your bhajis are cooked.

Add the remaining bhaji ingredients to the onion and carrot (except the vegetable oil), and mix together well. You want a sticky mixture. If it's too watery, add more chickpea flour.

If you're baking your bhajis, line a baking tray with greaseproof paper. Using your hands (it's much easier), grab about a tablespoon of the mixture and form into a small ball. After shaping place the balls straight onto the baking tray and bake for 15–20 minutes, or until golden and crisp. Turn the bhajis halfway through cooking.

If you're frying the bhajis, cook them in the prepared fryer, in batches, for about 4 minutes.

Once cooked, lightly season with salt to keep them crisp and serve with the mint yogurt.

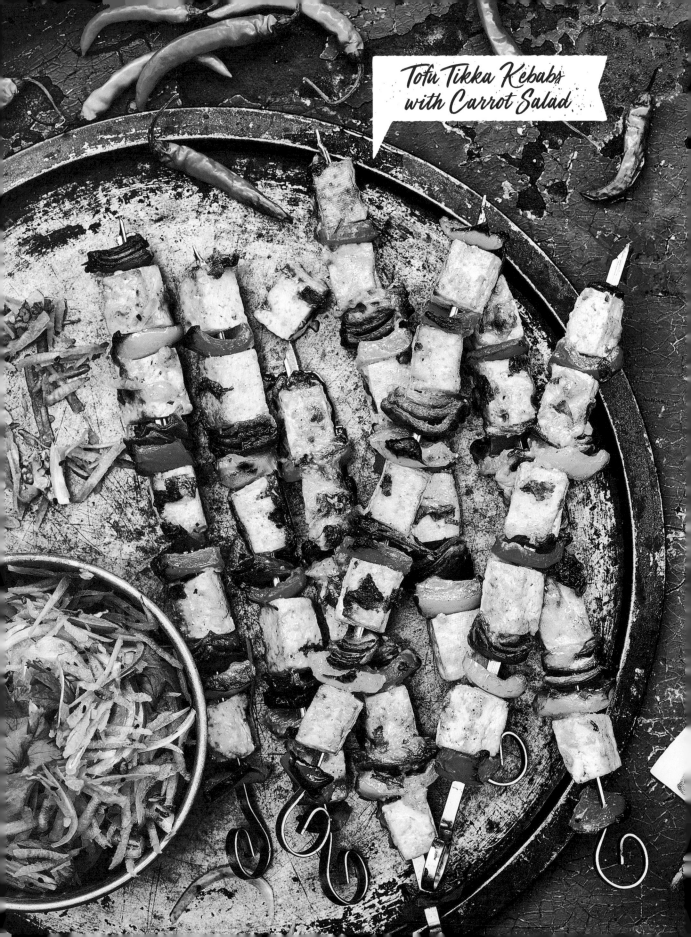

*Tofu Tikka Kebabs
with Carrot Salad*

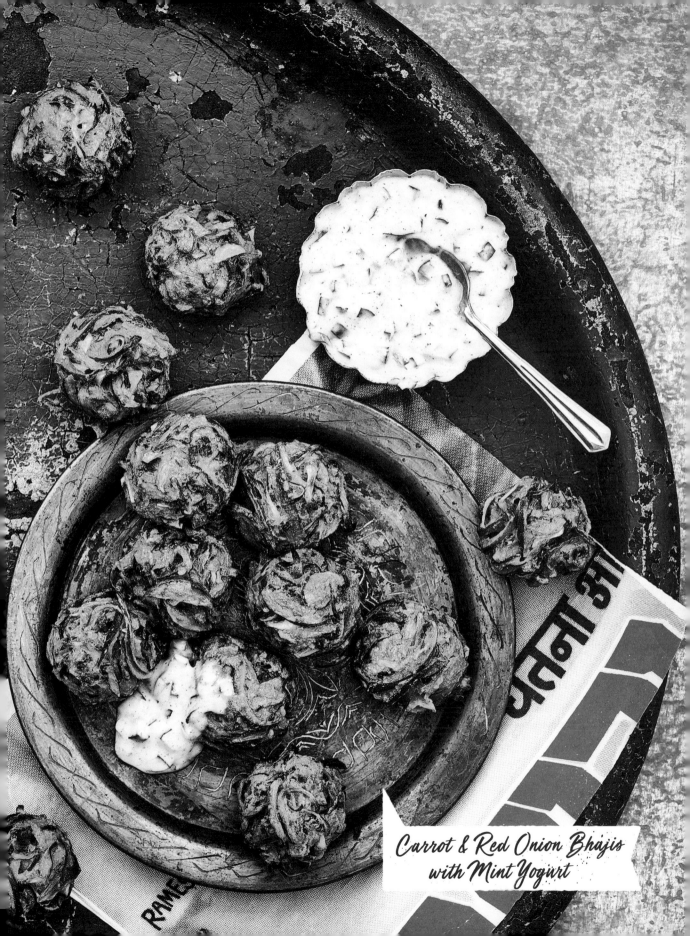

Carrot & Red Onion Bhajis with Mint Yogurt

GAZ'S "GUAC"

I could live off guacamole. I've added a slight twist to my classic guacamole with charred pepper, chilli and mango. The smoky charred flavour works so well with the creamy avocado. Don't cook the pepper, mango or chilli if you want to keep this dish raw.

SERVES 5–6

1 yellow (bell) pepper

1 tbsp extra virgin olive oil

1/2 mango, peeled

1 mild red chilli

2 ripe avocados

1 small red onion, finely chopped

6 cherry tomatoes, finely chopped

handful of fresh coriander (cilantro), chopped

juice of 1 lime

pinch sea salt and pepper

Light a small gas ring on your hob, place the pepper directly onto the flame and allow to char on all sides, using heatproof tongs to turn the pepper. Once charred, transfer to a sealable sandwich bag or a bowl and cover with cling film (plastic wrap). Set aside for 5 minutes while you prepare the rest of the ingredients. If you don't have a gas hob, simply place the pepper in a hot oven for 15 minutes.

Preheat a griddle pan over a high heat and add the oil, then grill the mango and chilli for 2–3 minutes. Try to add a little charring to the mango – the sugars caramelize and add a beautiful flavour.

Remove the flesh from the avocados and place in a large bowl with the red onion, tomatoes, coriander, lime and seasoning.

Mash it together, or use a stick blender to whizz until creamy. I like the odd lump in my guac.

Remove the pepper from the bag or bowl. Deseed and remove the stalk. Using the back of your knife, peel/scrape the charred skin away from the pepper flesh and discard. Finely chop the flesh and add it to the avocado mixture.

Finely chop the mango and chilli, then add to the bowl and give everything a good mix. Check the seasoning, then serve. Eat straight away.

HUMMUS 3 WAYS

I hope my hummus recipes will show you how simple it is to switch up classic hummus and make it even more delicious. All of these will keep in the fridge for up to 2 days.

ALL SERVE 4

SUPER PINK BEETROOT

1 x 400-g (14-oz) can chickpeas, drained and rinsed

3 garlic cloves

2 medium beetroots (beets), baked until soft

juice of 1 lemon

2 tbsp tahini

3 tbsp extra virgin olive oil, plus extra to serve

pinch salt and pepper

2–3 tbsp water or chickpea water

2 tbsp mixed seeds

Put all the ingredients except the seeds into a blender and blitz until smooth. Top with mixed seeds and a drizzle of olive oil.

PUMPKIN & SAGE

1 x 400-g (14-oz) can chickpeas, drained and rinsed

3 garlic cloves

200g (1 cup) cooked and chopped pumpkin flesh

juice of 1 lemon

1 tbsp dried sage

2 tbsp tahini

3 tbsp extra virgin olive oil

pinch salt and pepper

2–3 tbsp water or chickpea water

a few sage leaves, fried in a little oil (optional)

2 tbsp toasted pine nuts (optional)

Put all the ingredients except the sage leaves and pine nuts into a blender and blitz until smooth. Top with crispy sage leaves and toasted pine nuts if liked.

PAPRIKA & THYME

1 x 400-g (14-oz) can chickpeas, drained and rinsed

3 garlic cloves

juice and zest of 1 lemon

1 tbsp fresh thyme leaves, plus extra to serve

2 tsp smoked paprika

2 tbsp tahini

3 tbsp extra virgin olive oil

pinch salt and pepper

2–3 tbsp water or chickpea water

Put all the ingredients into a blender and blitz until smooth. Top with a sprinkle of paprika and fresh thyme leaves.

PERI PERI FALAFEL WITH TAHINI DRESSING

Herby, hearty and healthy... I have a slight addiction to falafel, but I think a lot of vegans do. Here, the traditional recipe is given a little twist.

MAKES ABOUT 15

For the falafel:

3 tbsp olive oil

1 onion, very finely chopped

3 garlic cloves, crushed

1 tbsp ground cumin

1 tsp smoked paprika

$\frac{1}{4}$ tsp ground ginger

1 tsp cayenne pepper

1 tsp dried oregano

480g (3 cups) canned chickpeas, drained and rinsed

handful of fresh coriander (cilantro), roughly chopped

zest and juice of $\frac{1}{2}$ lemon

3 tbsp buckwheat flour

$\frac{1}{2}$ tsp sea salt and pepper

For the tahini dressing:

1 tbsp tahini

5 tbsp cold filtered water

1 garlic clove, crushed

juice of $\frac{1}{2}$ lemon

pinch salt and pepper

$\frac{1}{4}$ tsp smoked paprika

To serve:

salad (any from the Salads chapter)

Grilled Flatbreads (see page 178)

Preheat the oven to 180°C (350°F) and line a baking tray with greaseproof paper.

First off, heat a non-stick frying pan over a medium heat. Add 1 tablespoon of the olive oil and add the chopped onion, garlic and spices. Sauté for 2–3 minutes, stirring often. I fry the onions and garlic with the spices and oregano first just to activate all the flavours.

Once the onions are soft and smelling beautiful, add them to your blender with the remaining falafel ingredients. Pop the lid on and blend until everything is chopped up nicely and starts to come together. You may have to scrape down the sides of the blender with a spatula a couple of times before you reach this point.

If your mixture is still crumbly and not combining, simply add more flour and oil, then blitz a little longer.

The best way to ball up your super-green falafel mix is using a melon baller; if you don't have one of those just roll equal quantities in your hands into balls.

Pop the falafels onto the tray and into the oven to bake for 15 minutes.

Meanwhile, make the dressing: simply add everything to a bowl and whisk until creamy.

Serve the falafel with the dressing, salad and flatbreads.

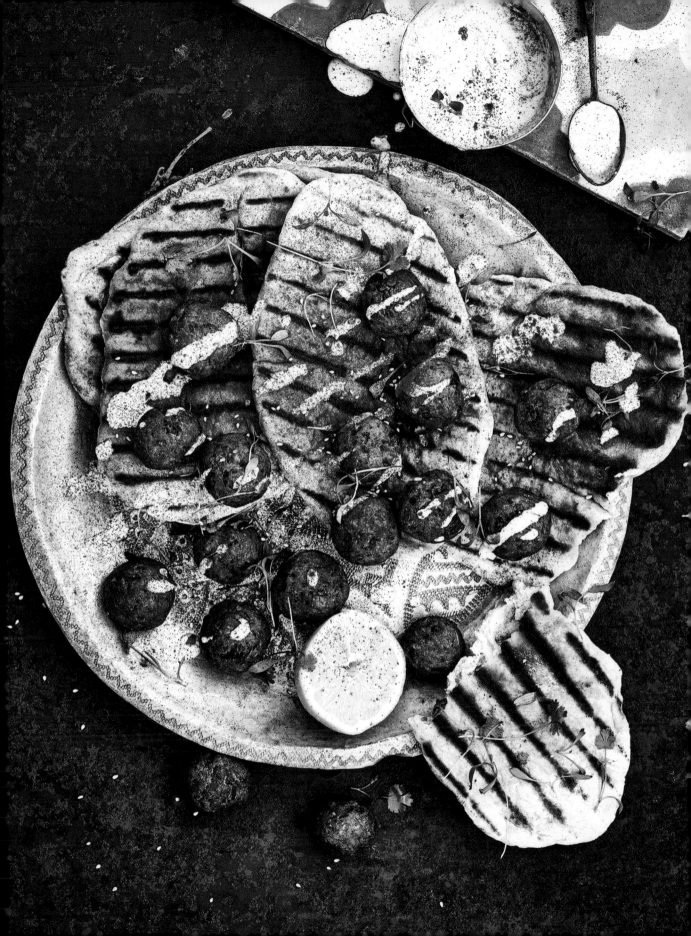

ROASTED BALSAMIC BEETROOT & SHALLOT TARTS

Beetroot and balsamic are a match made in heaven, and with my flaky puff pastry they're incredible. Add some of my "Cream Cheese" from page 15 for an extra delight.

SERVES 4 GENEROUSLY

5 beetroots (beets), peeled and sliced into 1-cm ($^3/_8$-inch) discs

6 shallots, peeled and halved lengthways

4 sprigs fresh thyme

3 tbsp balsamic vinegar

2 tbsp extra virgin olive oil

pinch sea salt and pepper

400g (14oz) Rough Puff Pastry (see page 30), or shop-bought vegan puff pastry

40g ($^1/_2$ cup) walnuts

3 tbsp "Cream Cheese" (see page 15)

fresh rocket (arugula), to serve

For the pastry glaze:

2 tsp agave nectar

2 tbsp extra virgin olive oil

2 tbsp almond Milk (see page 12)

Preheat the oven to 180°C (350°F) and line 2 baking trays with greaseproof paper.

Place the beetroot slices, shallots and thyme on one of the baking trays. Drizzle over the vinegar and olive oil, then season. Mix it all together so that everything is coated, then bake in the oven for 30–35 minutes, or until the vegetables are tender.

Meanwhile, prepare your pastry. It's up to you what size your tart will be but I like to make 2 big ones. Roll the pastry into a large rectangle around 3mm ($^1/_8$ inch) thick. Cut the pastry into two neat rectangles around 15 x 20cm (6 x 8 inches). Transfer the pastry onto the baking tray and lightly score a rough border with a sharp knife, approximately 2cm ($^3/_4$ inch) from the edge, all the way round. Prick over the middle with a fork, leaving the border untouched.

Midway through cooking the beetroot, place the pastry sheet/s into the oven on the shelf below, to lightly cook for 8–10 minutes. The border should puff up nicely.

Once the pastry and vegetables are cooked, use a palette knife to neatly place the beetroot and shallots in the middle of the pastry, then sprinkle over the walnuts and cheese.

Mix the ingredients for the pastry glaze together in a small bowl and brush over the pastry around the border.

Transfer the tarts back into the oven to cook for a further 10 minutes, until beautiful and golden. Serve with a little rocket sprinkled on top.

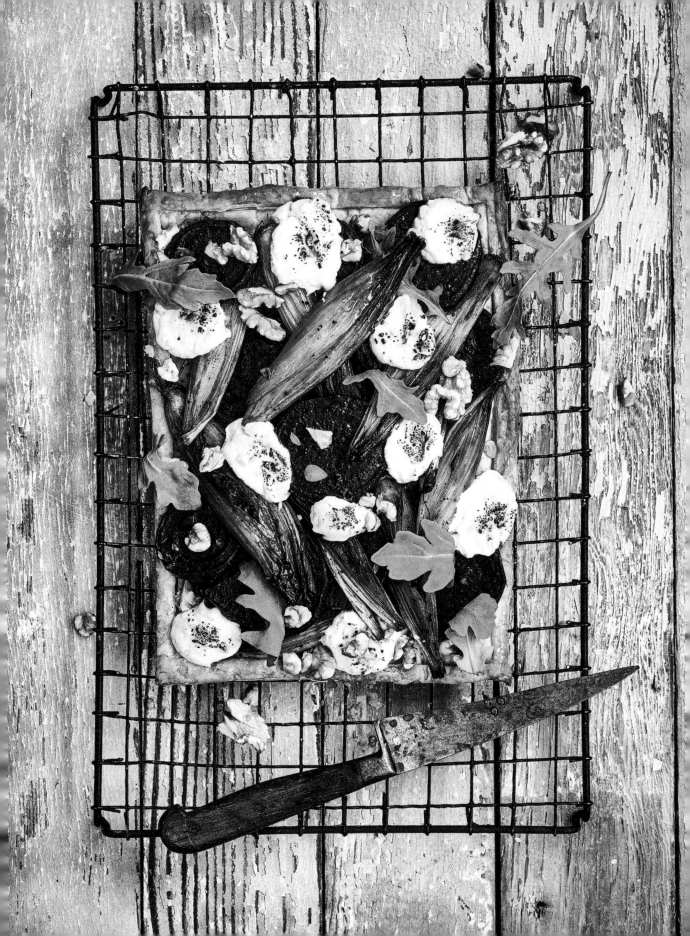

ULTIMATE VEGAN BAGUETTES

These are fully loaded subs that literally have a bit of everything in – your taste buds will be having a party! I've added a quick Asian-inspired dressing to the tofu. It works really well with the fresh vegetables and pickled onion and radish. You can make these ahead and take them to work with you; just make sure your grilled tofu is cool before filling the baguette if you aren't eating it right away.

SERVES 2

200g (7oz) firm tofu, drained and thinly sliced

2 small baguettes or sub-rolls

1 carrot, sliced into ribbons

10-cm (4-inch) piece of cucumber, sliced into ribbons

2 spring onions (scallions), finely sliced

handful of fresh coriander (cilantro)

For the dressing:

2 tbsp soy sauce

2 tbsp sesame oil

juice of $\frac{1}{2}$ lime

1 tsp dried chilli flakes

2 tsp maple syrup or agave nectar

$\frac{1}{2}$ tsp ginger, finely chopped

pinch garlic powder

For the pickled onion and radish:

$\frac{1}{2}$ red onion, sliced into rings

8 radishes, finely sliced

3 tbsp rice vinegar

1 tsp coconut sugar

pinch sea salt

First up, mix together all the dressing ingredients in a small mixing bowl, leaving 1 tablespoon of the oil aside for frying. Add the tofu slices, then set aside for 5 minutes.

Put all the pickled onion and radish ingredients with 2 tbsp water in another bowl, stir to combine and leave to lightly pickle.

Preheat a griddle pan over a high heat and add the reserved oil. Grill the tofu slices until lightly charred on each side. Brush over more of the dressing while cooking.

Fill your baguettes or rolls with the chargrilled tofu, carrot and cucumber ribbons, spring onion and coriander, then top with some of the beautiful pickled onion and radish, and enjoy.

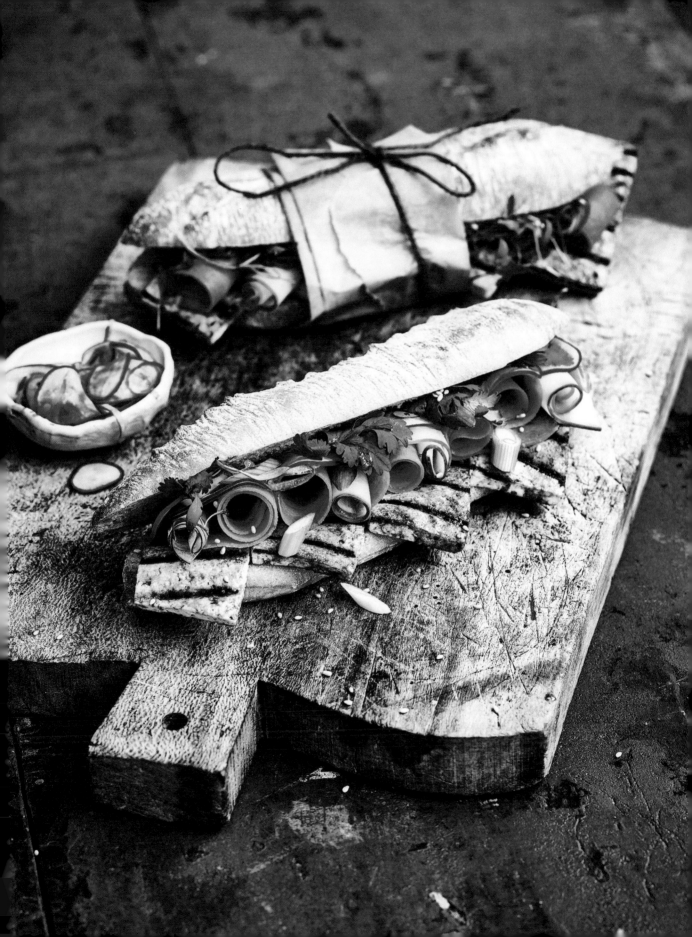

SPICY SWEETCORN & KALE POTATO RÖSTI WITH MANGO SALSA

These rösti are seriously good, and pan-frying them in coconut oil adds a really golden crispness. They are ready within 30 minutes, too!

MAKES ABOUT 6

2 large Maris Piper potatoes, peeled

165g (1 cup) cooked sweetcorn kernels

130g (1 cup) steamed and finely shredded kale

3 spring onions (scallions), very finely chopped

1 medium red chilli, deseeded and finely chopped

handful of coriander (cilantro), finely chopped

4 tbsp plain (all-purpose) flour or buckwheat flour

2 tbsp Egg Replacement (see page 32)

2 tbsp extra virgin olive oil

1 tsp paprika

1 tsp cayenne pepper

1 tbsp lime juice

pinch sea salt and pepper

1 tbsp coconut oil, for frying

For the mango salsa:

1 ripe mango, chopped into small cubes

1 red chilli, deseeded and finely chopped

1 red onion, finely chopped

2 tomatoes, deseeded and finely chopped

handful of fresh coriander (cilantro), finely chopped

juice of 1 lime

pinch sea salt

Preheat the oven to 180°C (350°F), line a baking tray with greaseproof paper and dust with a little flour.

First make the salsa: simply stir everything together in a mixing bowl, cover with cling film (plastic wrap) and refrigerate until ready to serve.

Now make the rösti. Grab yourself a big mixing bowl and grate the potatoes into it. Tip the grated potato into the centre of a clean tea towel, gather up each corner then twist the tea towel over the sink to squeeze out as much of the liquid as possible.

Tip the drained potato back into the mixing bowl and add the other rösti ingredients. Stir together until everything is well incorporated. The mixture should be quite sticky and start to come together. If not, add a touch more flour and olive oil or egg replacer.

Form discs with around 2 tbsp rösti mixture in your hands, then place them onto the lined, dusted baking tray. You can make them a little neater on the tray.

Preheat a large, non-stick frying pan over a low heat, then add a little coconut oil.

A few at a time, add the rösti to the frying pan and fry until golden on each side. This should take no longer than 3–4 minutes. Place them back onto the tray. Repeat until you've fried all the rösti, then transfer the tray to the oven and bake for 15 minutes.

Once the rösti are cooked and nicely golden, remove from the oven and serve straight away with the mango salsa.

SUMMER ROLLS WITH SWEET CHILLI DIP

These rolls are tasty, nourishing and beautiful to look at. When I make these, I know summer has arrived. You can fill them with whatever you like but make sure you try my raw sweet chilli dip – it's the perfect dipping sauce for summer rolls.

MAKES 10

For the summer rolls:

10 rice paper wraps

1/2 fennel bulb, finely shredded

1 courgette (zucchini), cut into fine batons

1 carrot, peeled and cut into fine batons

1 beetroot (beet), peeled and cut into fine discs

10-cm (4-inch) piece of cucumber, deseeded and cut into fine batons

handful of mint leaves

1 kiwi, peeled and finely sliced

12 baby gem lettuce leaves, shredded

handful of Thai basil

handful of raw peanuts

For the sweet chilli dip:

4 tbsp apple cider vinegar

3 tsp lime juice

2 tbsp coconut sugar or maple syrup

4 tsp sun-dried tomato paste

1 tsp dried chilli flakes

2 tsp sesame seeds

pinch sea salt

First make the dip: throw everything into a mixing bowl with 3 tbsp water and whisk together. Cover the bowl with cling film (plastic wrap), then place in the fridge until ready to serve.

Next up, the beautiful rice paper rolls. Fill a small bowl full of warm water and individually dip the rice paper wraps into the water until they are pliable.

When pliable, fill them with the prepared vegetables, herbs, kiwi and nuts. Fill them as full as you can. I like to add a little drizzle of the sweet chilli dip in the middle before rolling them.

Once you've rolled them all up, serve chilled with the sweet chilli dip on the side. Delightful!

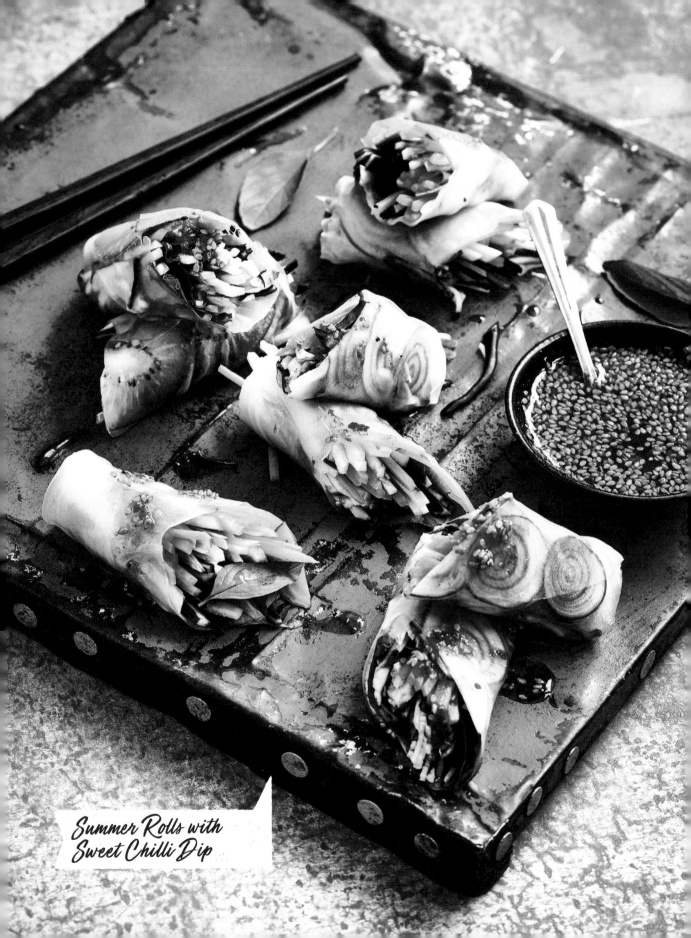

*Summer Rolls with
Sweet Chilli Dip*

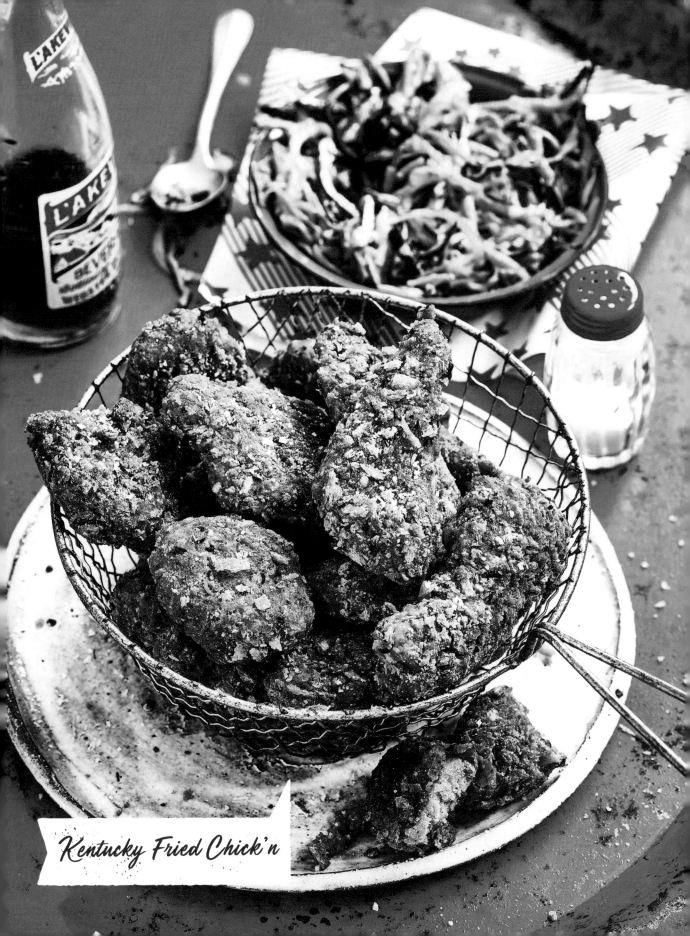

Kentucky Fried Chick'n

KENTUCKY FRIED CHICK'N

These seitan chick'n pieces are tender as hell! I coat them in a wonderful spicy batter that will rival any. They become super-crispy if fried but you can also bake them. If you are short of time you can also use the same batter technique with cauliflower florets.

SERVES 4

For the chick'n – wet:

170g (1 cup) firm tofu

120ml (1/2 cup) soy milk

1 tsp miso paste

1 tsp dried tarragon

1 tsp dried sage

1/2 tsp onion powder

1/4 tsp garlic powder

1 tsp sea salt

For the chick'n – dry:

115g (1 cup) seitan
(vital wheat gluten)

25g (1/4 cup) chickpea (gram) flour

For the broth:

1 litre (4 cups) Vegetable Stock (see page 31)

1 sprig fresh rosemary

2 sprigs fresh thyme

1 onion, quartered

pinch sea salt and pepper

For the Kentucky coating:

120g (1 cup) plain
(all-purpose) flour

60g (1 cup) panko breadcrumbs

2 tbsp unrefined caster
(superfine) sugar

1 tsp sea salt

2 tsp cracked black pepper

1 tbsp cayenne pepper

1 tbsp dried chilli flakes

1 tbsp dried oregano

1 tbsp paprika

1 tbsp dried sage

1 tsp ground allspice

For the batter:

100g (1 cup) chickpea (gram) flour

240ml (1 cup) water

1 litre (4 cups) vegetable oil, for frying

First up, you will need to make the chick'n pieces. Combine all the wet ingredients in a blender and blitz until smooth.

Put the dry ingredients in a large mixing bowl and mix well.

Add the wet mix to the bowl and stir until the mixture forms a dough. Turn the dough out onto a clean work surface lightly floured with chickpea flour.

Knead the dough for at least 8 minutes. This is the most important part of the recipe. If you don't knead it properly, you will be left with horrible, spongy seitan. (I have gone as far as pounding the seitan dough with my fists!)

Once kneaded, the dough will be quite firm and elastic. Form it into a rectangle around 1cm ($^3/_8$ inch) thick and cut it into 4. Set aside to rest for 10 minutes whilst you prepare the cooking broth.

Add all the broth ingredients to a large, lidded saucepan and bring to a boil, then turn the heat down so that the broth is just lightly simmering.

Add the seitan pieces to the broth and pop the lid on. Simmer the seitan pieces for 35 minutes in the simmering broth (do not let it boil). Flip the seitan pieces over halfway through cooking.

After the 35 minutes, remove the seitan pieces from the broth and set aside to cool. They should have almost doubled in size and feel quite meaty. Once cool, tear or cut them into smaller pieces ready to be covered in the Kentucky coating. I like to tear the pieces as this creates rough edges for the coating to cling on to.

For the Kentucky coating, stir all the ingredients together in a mixing bowl.

For the batter, mix the chickpea flour and water together in a separate bowl.

Now it's time to individually dip the seitan pieces – first into the chickpea batter then into the coating. I double dip them to make sure they have a nice thick coating. Once you've coated all of the pieces, put them on a plate in the fridge while you heat the oil.

If you're using a deep-fat fryer, set it to 180°C (350°F). Alternatively, pour the oil into a large saucepan but don't fill it more than half full.

To test if the oil is hot enough in the saucepan, drop a cube of bread into the oil – if it floats to the top straight away, the oil is ready. Carefully fry the chick'n pieces for 3–4 minutes, or until golden and crisp.

If you'd prefer to bake the chick'n pieces, bake for 25 minutes in an oven set at 180°C (350°F).

Once cooked, transfer to a plate lined with kitchen paper to soak up any excess oil. Serve immediately.

BURGERS, DOGS & WRAPS

KATSU TOFU BURGER

This is everything I love inside a burger – the crispy tofu is incredible! Huge crunches when you eat this. You don't have to deep-fry the tofu; baking works just as well. Keep it gluten free by swapping the breadcrumbs, flour and bun for g-f alternatives.

MAKES 4 BURGERS

For the tofu:

4 tbsp cornflour (cornstarch)

50g (1 cup) panko breadcrumbs

4 tbsp plain (all-purpose) flour

400g (14oz) firm tofu, drained and cut into 4 "steaks"

1 litre (4 cups) vegetable oil, if frying

For the curried mayo:

6 tbsp Creamy "Mayonnaise" (see page 24)

1 tsp curry powder

1/4 tsp dried chilli powder

1/4 tsp black onion seeds

2 tsp lemon juice

pinch sea salt

To serve:

4 burger buns, toasted

8 baby gem lettuce leaves

pickled onion and radish (see page 92)

3 spring onions (scallions), chopped

fresh coriander (cilantro)

Heat your fryer to 170°C (340°F) or, if baking, preheat the oven to 180°C (350°F).

First up, prepare the tofu. Mix the cornflour in a bowl with enough water to make a thick, sticky paste. Put the breadcrumbs in a shallow bowl and the plain flour in another.

Individually, dip each tofu steak first into the flour, then the cornflour paste (making sure it's well covered), then finally coat in the breadcrumbs. Once all pieces are coated, set aside.

Mix together all the mayo ingredients and prepare the burger garnishes.

To cook the burgers, carefully deep-fry in the oil until golden, then drain on kitchen paper and season.

Alternatively, bake on a lined baking tray for 15 minutes.

Once the tofu is cooked, build your burger, making sure you have lashings of curried mayonnaise and plenty of the garnishes.

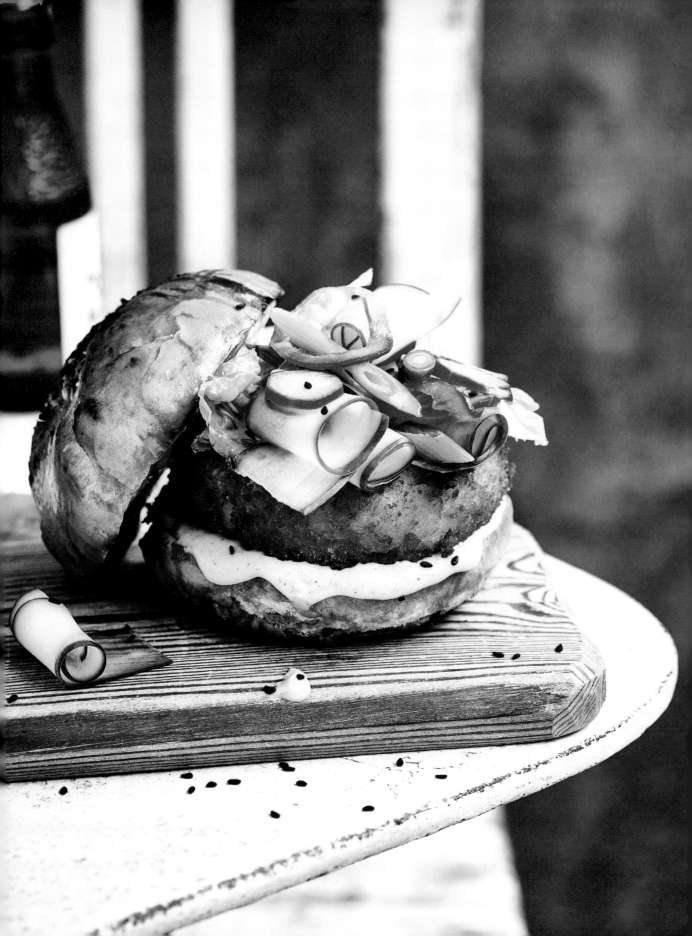

SMOKY CHICKPEA & GRILLED SQUASH FLATBREAD WRAPS

These smoky, delicious warming flavours work so well with the amazing grilled flatbreads for this dish, especially if they are still slightly warm.

MAKES 5

1 small butternut squash

1 tsp coconut oil

3–4 tbsp olive oil

1 red onion, finely sliced

250g (1¼ cups) canned chickpeas, drained and rinsed

1 tsp smoked paprika

¼ tsp cayenne pepper

¼ tsp ground cumin

2 sprigs fresh thyme

10 fresh sage leaves

juice of ½ lemon

pinch salt and pepper

To serve:

hummus (see page 87)

5 Grilled Flatbreads (see page 178) or wraps of your choice, warmed

100g (1 cup) finely shredded red cabbage

sprinkle of mixed seeds

First up, the butternut squash, as that takes the longest to cook. Split the squash in half at the point where the long "neck" meets the round base. Pop the base in your fridge for another use. Peel the "neck" with a peeler or serrated knife, then cut the flesh into evenly sized batons (approximately 2 x 10cm [¾ x 4 inches]), so they'll fit nicely in the wrap.

Tip the squash batons into a saucepan of cold water, then place over a medium heat for approximately 10 minutes, or until the batons are just cooked through. Be careful not to over-cook as they will be grilled later. Drain away the water.

Preheat a griddle pan and a non-stick frying pan. Add a little coconut oil to the griddle pan, and the olive oil to the frying pan. Once the griddle pan is hot, add the squash and lightly grill on all sides. Sprinkle over some seasoning while it's cooking.

Add the onion to the frying pan. When soft, add the chickpeas and the spices, stirring often. After 2 minutes, add the fresh thyme and sage leaves: try to let the sage crisp up nicely. Cook for another minute then add the lemon juice for some freshness. Sprinkle over some seasoning and remove from the heat.

To serve, spoon a generous amount of hummus onto the slightly warm wraps, then add the grilled squash followed by the smoky chickpea mix. Make sure each wrap has a few of the beautiful crispy sage leaves. Add a small handful of shredded red cabbage for that vibrant colour and fresh peppery flavour, then finish with a sprinkle of seeds.

KENTUCKY BBQ PULLED JACKFRUIT & SHIITAKE LETTUCE WRAPS

Jackfruit is a wonder-fruit – highly nutritious with a surprisingly meaty texture – and is often compared to pulled pork! Covered in a sticky, smoky BBQ sauce, coupled with shiitake mushrooms and wrapped in lettuce wraps, it tastes amazing.

MAKES 5

2 x 400-g (14-oz) cans young jackfruit in water/brine

1 tsp fennel seeds, toasted and ground

1 tsp dried sage

1 tsp smoked paprika

1 tsp cayenne pepper

1 tsp ground cumin

1 tsp sugar

1 tbsp coconut oil

1 red onion, finely chopped

120g (1½ cups) shiitake mushrooms, hard stalks removed and thinly sliced

240g (1 cup) BBQ Sauce (see page 24)

To serve:

4 heads baby gem lettuce

Rainbow Slaw (see page 162)

toasted cashew nuts

First up, drain the jackfruit and pat dry with kitchen paper. You will see that the jackfruit is cut into triangle shapes – remove the hard core, then using your hands break the tender bits into a mixing bowl. You will come across some seeds; discard those as well.

Once you have all the tender stringy bits in your bowl, add the herbs, spices and sugar. Give it a really good mix so that each piece of jackfruit is coated.

Next heat a large, non-stick frying pan over a medium heat. Add the coconut oil followed by the onions and mushrooms. Cook for 3 minutes, stirring constantly.

Try and get the mushrooms and onions really golden and caramelized as this will add great flavour.

Once they are golden, add the seasoned jackfruit and sauté for 2–3 minutes, adding some good colour and letting the sugar caramelize nicely.

Add the BBQ sauce, give it a good stir, then reduce the heat. Cook for 8–10 minutes over a low heat, stirring often.

To serve, place the sautéed BBQ jackfruit inside your lettuce leaves, topped with rainbow slaw and toasted cashews.

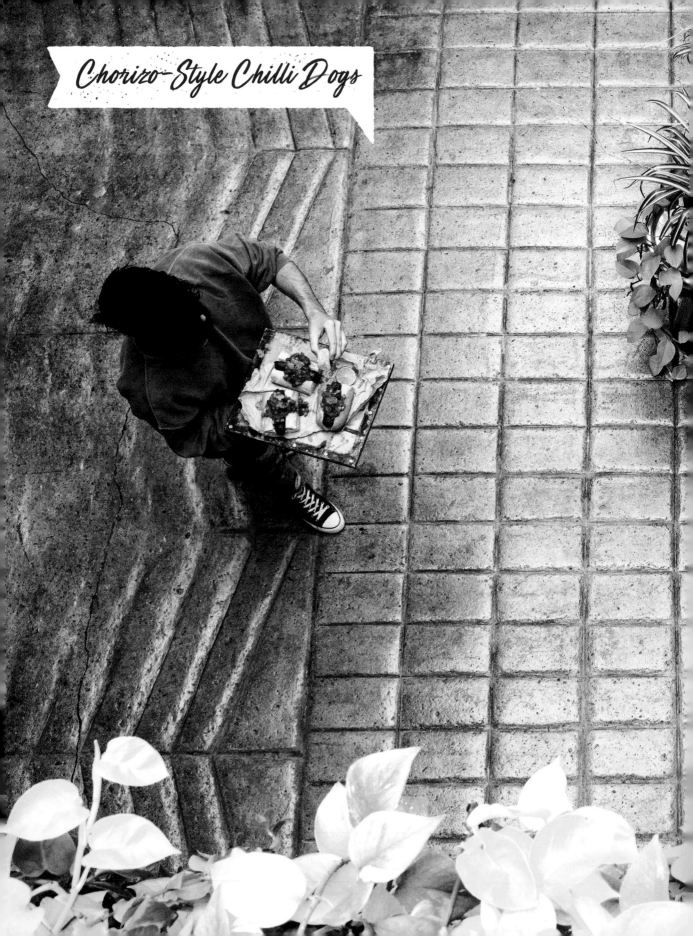

Chorizo-Style Chilli Dogs

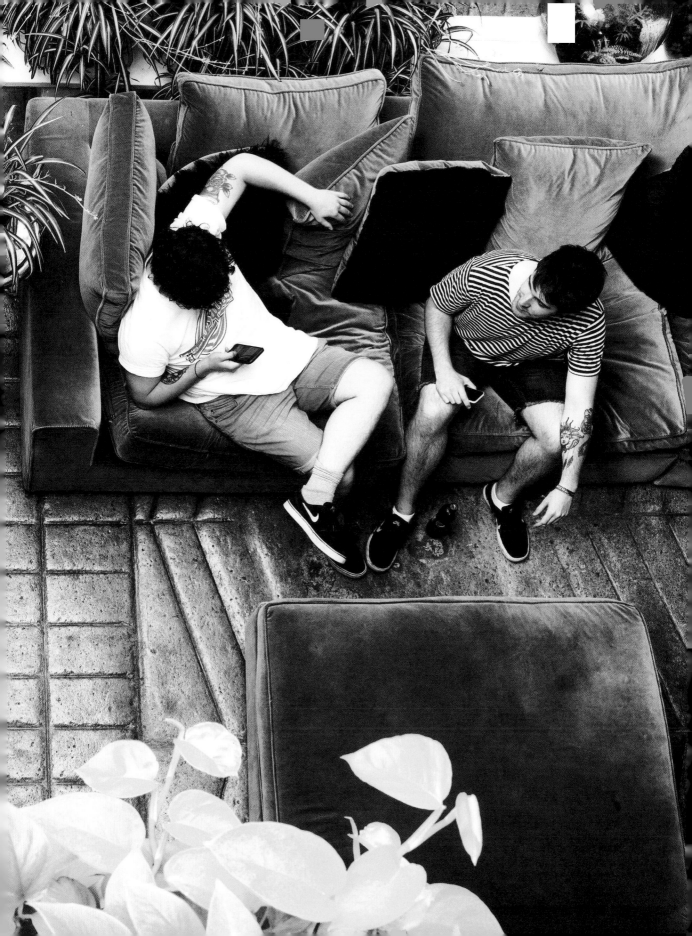

CHORIZO-STYLE CHILLI DOGS

Here is another seitan treat packed full of those classic chorizo flavours, such as smoked paprika and fennel seeds. I like to top my sausages with a spicy chilli (which is just as nice with a bowl of rice and salad).

MAKES 8 SAUSAGES

For the sausages – wet:

290ml (1$\frac{1}{4}$ cups) hot Vegetable Stock (see page 31)

3 tbsp dried porcini mushrooms

a little coconut oil, for sautéing

1 medium red onion, peeled and roughly chopped

2 garlic cloves, crushed

1 tbsp extra virgin olive oil

100g ($\frac{1}{2}$ cup) canned chickpeas, drained and rinsed

4 tbsp tomato puree

2$\frac{1}{2}$ tbsp smoked paprika

1 tbsp cayenne pepper

1 tbsp fennel seeds

1 tsp salt and pepper

1 tbsp miso paste

For the sausages – dry:

270g (2$\frac{1}{3}$ cups) seitan (vital wheat gluten)

50g ($\frac{1}{2}$ cup) chickpea (gram) flour

2 tbsp nutritional yeast

For the chilli:

1 red onion, finely chopped

2 garlic cloves

1 fresh jalapeño chilli

1 small butternut squash, peeled and cut into small cubes

1 red (bell) pepper, cubed

a little coconut oil, for sautéing

1 tsp ground cumin

1 tsp ground cinnamon

2 tsp cayenne pepper

pinch sea salt and pepper

2 x 400-g (14-oz) cans chopped tomatoes

200g (1 cup) canned chickpeas, drained and rinsed

200g (1 cup) canned red kidney beans, drained and rinsed

100g ($\frac{1}{2}$ cup) sweetcorn, cooked

handful of chopped coriander (cilantro)

To serve:

hot dog rolls

avocado slices

"Crème Fraîche" (see page 17)

fresh coriander (cilantro)

[Continued on page 110...]

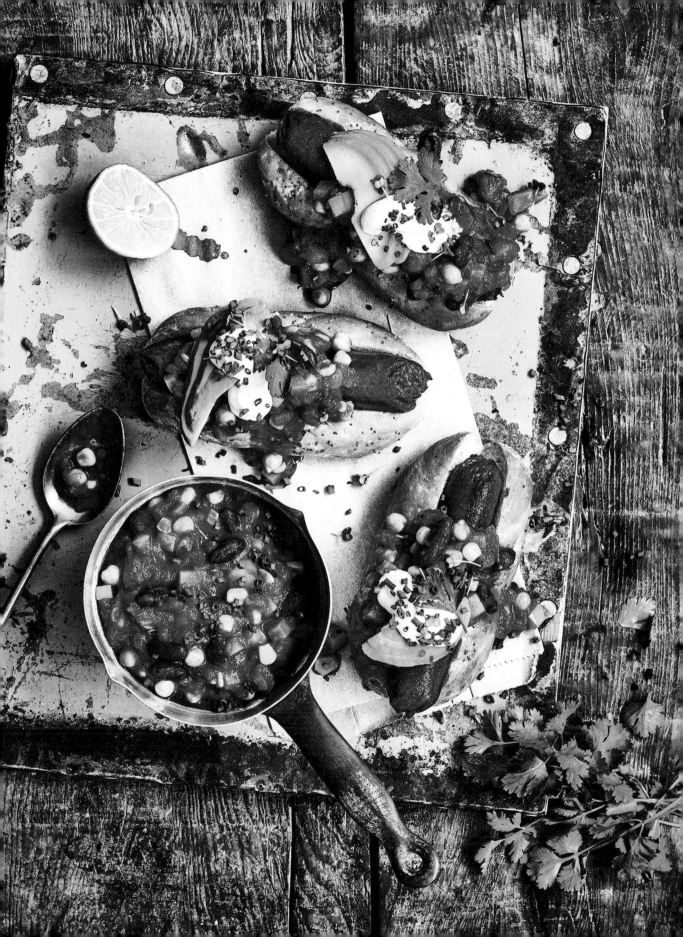

CHORIZO-STYLE CHILLI DOGS (CONT.)

First up, make the seitan "chorizo" sausages. Pour the hot vegetable stock onto the porcini in a bowl and set aside for 5 minutes for the porcini to rehydrate.

Heat a non-stick saucepan and add a touch of coconut oil. When the pan is hot, add the onions and garlic. Reduce the heat and allow them to soften and lightly caramelize for around 2 minutes, stirring often.

Remove the pan from the heat and tip the onions and garlic into a blender with the remaining wet ingredients, plus mushrooms and stock. Let the mixture sit for 5 minutes to cool slightly before you blitz, while you put all the dry ingredients into a large mixing bowl.

Blitz the wet mixture until smooth, then scrape the blended mixture into the dry ingredients and stir quickly with a spatula until everything is well combined.

You will now need to use your hands to knead the dough. Knead for around 10 minutes either in the bowl or on a clean work surface. Your dough will be quite wet so sprinkle a little chickpea flour onto the surface (or in the bowl). The tougher you are when kneading, the more of a bite/meat-like texture your sausages will have when cooked, so be firm! Once kneaded, divide the dough

into approximately 8 pieces. I weigh each piece to make sure all my sausages are a similar size – aim for around 110g (4oz).

Heat a large, lidded saucepan half full of water until boiling, then reduce the heat so that the water is at a rolling simmer.

Prepare 8 pieces of foil, shiny side up, approximately 25cm (10 inches) long. (If you don't like using foil, use greaseproof baking paper instead.) Dot a little oil onto the foil.

Roll a piece of dough into a sausage shape with your hands before rolling up in a piece of foil. Twist each end and set aside. Do this for the rest of the dough pieces, then wrap each sausage tightly in cling film (plastic wrap).

Lower the wrapped sausages into the saucepan, pop the lid on and simmer for 50 minutes. Don't let it boil – keep a constant slow simmer – and give them a little stir every now and then.

After the 50 minutes, the sausages should be firm to the touch. Lift one out and check – be careful because they will be very hot! If it is still soft pop it back in the water to cook for a further 10 minutes. Once cooked, lift the sausages out of the pan and onto a wire rack to cool a little. Once the sausages are

cool enough to handle, remove the wrapping and leave to cool completely before refrigerating until use (or freezing).

To make the chilli, sauté the onion, garlic, chilli, squash and pepper in a little coconut oil in a large saucepan for 2–3 minutes whilst stirring. Add all of the spices and sauté for a further 2 minutes.

Add some seasoning, then the chopped tomatoes. Stir to combine, then pop the lid on and turn the heat down low. Allow to simmer for 10 minutes.

After 10 minutes, add the chickpeas, beans, sweetcorn and coriander and stir together. Taste it to check if it needs more seasoning or spice. If you like your chilli slightly spicier, add another teaspoon of cayenne pepper.

Simmer for 6–8 more minutes or until the squash is cooked through.

When you are ready to eat... fry, grill, bake or BBQ the sausages for about 12 minutes until golden.

Serve inside hot dog rolls topped with a spoonful of the beautiful chilli, some avocado, crème fraîche and fresh coriander.

QUARTER POUNDERS

This is the "meatiest" vegan burger around – it's almost like a steak burger – but it's made with wheat gluten, or seitan, and is full of protein and packed with flavour. These can be grilled, fried and barbequed. The burgers are actually best made a day ahead as they'll firm up more, so I often make a batch of these and pop them in the fridge overnight. They also freeze well.

MAKES 6 BURGERS

For the burger – wet:

300ml (1¼ cups) hot Vegetable Stock (see page 31)

3 tbsp dried porcini mushrooms

a little coconut oil, for frying

1 red onion, finely chopped

2 garlic cloves, finely chopped

50g (½ cup) canned black beans

3 tbsp tomato puree

1 tbsp soy sauce

1 tbsp balsamic vinegar

1 tbsp brown rice miso paste

1 tbsp Marmite

1 tsp smoked paprika

1 tsp dried chives

1 tsp dried oregano

½ tsp dried rosemary

2 tsp dried chilli flakes

1 tsp sea salt

1 tbsp cracked black pepper

For the burger – dry:

270g (2⅓ cups) seitan (vital wheat gluten)

50g (½ cup) chickpea (gram) flour

1 tbsp nutritional yeast

For the broth:

1 litre (4 cups) Vegetable Stock (see page 31)

1 tbsp miso paste

1 onion, peeled and quartered

3 garlic cloves

2 sprigs rosemary

3 tbsp dried porcini mushrooms

To serve:

burger buns, toasted

Chipotle Burger "Cheese" Slices (see page 115)

Quick Onion Rings (see page 115)

baby gem lettuce leaves

tomato slices

Creamy "Mayonnaise" (see page 24)

Hot Pink Beetroot Ketchup (see page 25)

[Continued on page 114...]

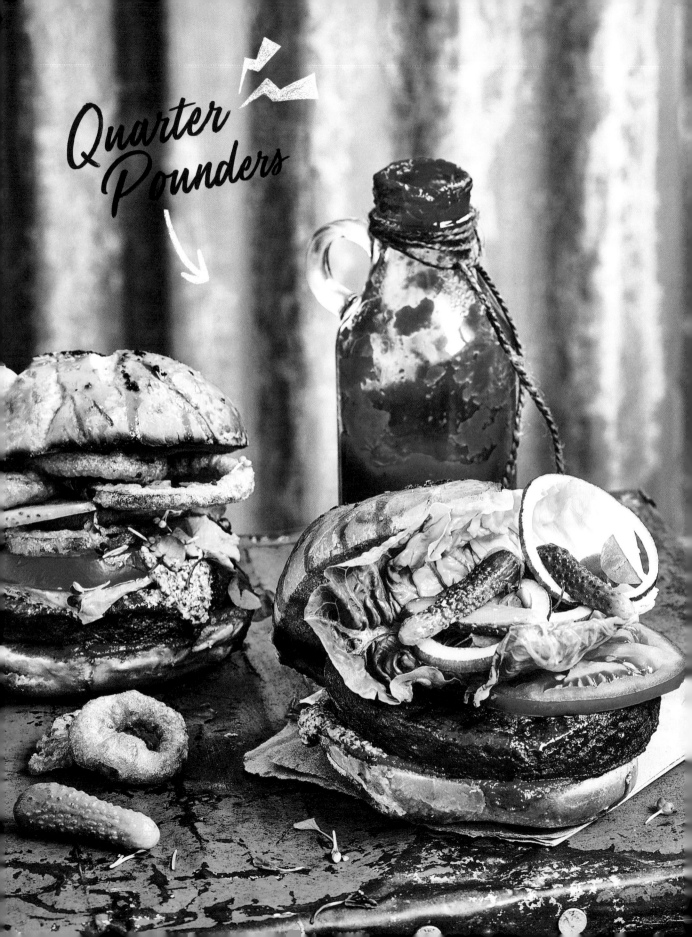

Quarter Pounders

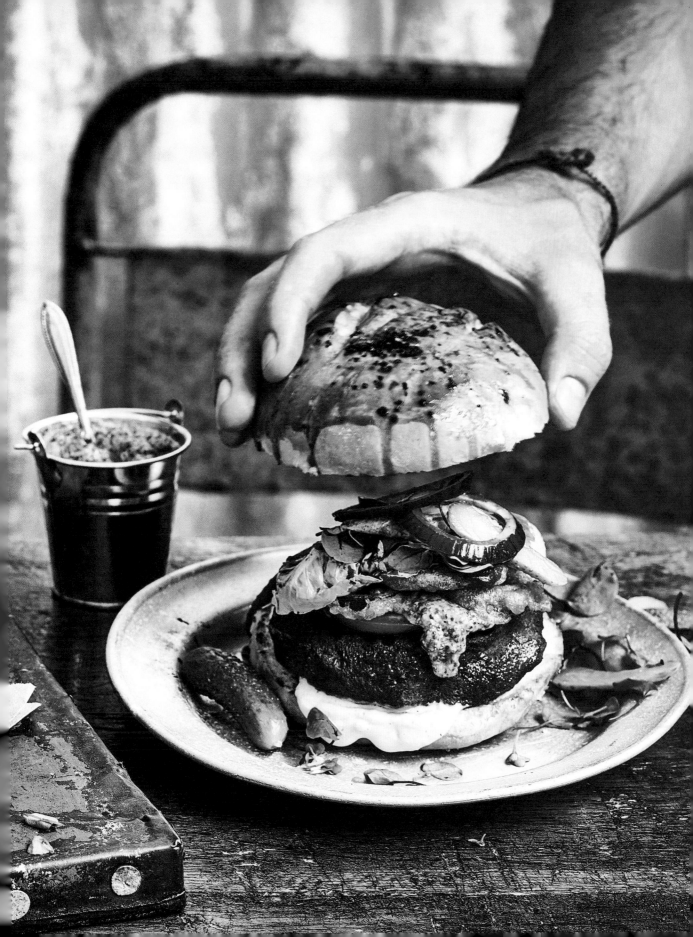

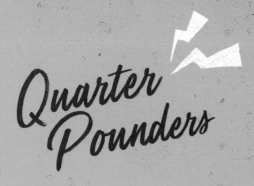

QUARTER POUNDERS (CONT.)

To make the burgers, first mix the hot vegetable stock with the porcini and set aside for 5 minutes for the porcini to rehydrate.

Heat a non-stick saucepan and add a touch of coconut oil. When the pan is hot, sauté the onions and garlic. Turn the heat down low and let them soften and lightly caramelize for around 2 minutes, stirring often.

Remove the pan from the heat and tip the onions and garlic into a blender with the remaining wet burger ingredients, plus the mushrooms and stock. Let the mixture sit for 5 minutes to cool slightly while you put the dry ingredients into a large bowl.

Blitz the wet mixture until smooth, then scrape the wet mixture into the mixing bowl with the dry ingredients and quickly stir with a spatula until everything is well combined and forms a dough.

You'll need to use your hands to knead the dough for 10 minutes in the bowl or on a clean work surface. The dough may be quite wet so sprinkle a little chickpea flour on the surface. It's important to knead well – the tougher you are when kneading, the more of a bite/meat-like texture your burgers will have when cooked, so be firm! After kneading, pop the dough back in the bowl, cover with a clean tea towel and set aside to rest and firm up for 15 minutes.

While the dough is resting, prepare the broth ingredients and put them all into a large, lidded saucepan (it needs to fit the burgers in) and slowly heat to a boil.

While the broth is heating up, it's time to form the dough into patties. The easiest way to do this is to roll the dough out with a rolling pin to no more than 2cm ($^3/_4$ inch) thick (the burgers expand when cooking). The dough will be quite tough to roll, so put your back into it! Once your dough is rolled out, use an 11-cm (4-inch) plain cookie cutter to cut your dough into burger shapes.

The broth should be boiling by now, so reduce to a rolling simmer. Carefully lower the burgers into the broth using a fish slice and cover the saucepan. Simmer over a low heat for 55 minutes, stirring a couple of times while the burgers are cooking.

After 55 minutes, turn the heat off and let the broth cool for 10 minutes before removing the now firm burgers. At this point you can either wait for the burgers to cool, then refrigerate for use the following day, or freeze, or you can cook them straight away.

My favourite method is to grill the burgers over a high heat for 15 minutes, turning halfway. I love the chargrilled lines and flavour.

Serve the burgers in a bun, with chipotle burger cheese slices, onion rings, lettuce, tomato, mayonnaise and/or my favourite beetroot ketchup.

CHIPOTLE BURGER "CHEESE" SLICES

These smoky chipotle "cheese" slices are the perfect accompaniment to my seitan quarter pounder burgers!

240ml (1 cup) soy milk

2 tsp chipotle paste

3 tbsp nutritional yeast

3 tbsp plain (all-purpose) flour

3 tsp agar agar powder

1 tsp miso paste

$\frac{1}{4}$ tsp mustard powder

$\frac{1}{4}$ tsp onion powder

1 tsp liquid smoke (optional)

$\frac{1}{2}$ tsp sea salt

Line a large baking tray with cling film (plastic wrap).

Put all the ingredients into a blender and blitz until smooth.

Pour the mixture into a non-stick saucepan over a low heat and whisk until it thickens. After about a minute start stirring with a spatula. Keep stirring until it's super-thick – this should only take 2–3 minutes in total.

Remove from the heat then quickly pour onto the lined tray. Use a palette knife to spread it out evenly to about 2mm ($\frac{1}{16}$ inch) thick, then pop the tray into the fridge to set for around 2 hours.

To serve, cut the cheese into squares and pop on top of your burger! I like doing this when the burger is cooking, either in the pan or oven, so the cheese melts beautifully.

QUICK ONION RINGS

Here's my quick and simple recipe for the crispiest onion rings.

120g (1 cup) plain (all-purpose) flour

2 tbsp white wine vinegar

180ml ($\frac{3}{4}$ cup) sparkling water

pinch sea salt and pepper

1 large red onion, peeled and sliced into rings

750ml (3 cups) vegetable oil, for frying

Whisk together the flour, vinegar, water and seasoning in a large mixing bowl. Preheat your fryer to 180°C (350°F) (or half-fill a large saucepan with the vegetable oil and heat up – it will be ready to use when a piece of bread carefully dropped in rises to the surface immediately and starts to sizzle).

Individually, dip the onion rings into the batter then carefully lower them into the fryer or saucepan.

Only fry 3–4 at a time for around 4 minutes, or until golden. Transfer to a plate lined with kitchen paper to drain off the excess oil. Continue until all the onion rings are fried and eat straight away.

THE MEXICAN

Classic Mexican flavours are jam-packed into this burger – it's a winner!
There's also a great mix of pulses, so it's very nutritious, and it's gluten free.

MAKES 4 BURGERS

For the burger:

200g (1 cup) chickpeas

90g ($\frac{1}{2}$ cup) red kidney beans

80g ($\frac{1}{2}$ cup) black beans

200g (1 cup) sweetcorn

2 spring onions (scallions),
finely chopped

1 small red chilli, finely chopped

handful of coriander (cilantro)

1 tbsp chipotle paste

5 tbsp buckwheat flour

zest and juice of $\frac{1}{2}$ lime

1 tbsp Cajun spice

2 tbsp extra virgin olive oil

a little coconut oil for frying

For the tomato salsa:

2 ripe tomatoes, finely sliced

handful of fresh coriander (cilantro)

$\frac{1}{2}$ red onion, sliced into fine rings

1 fresh jalapeño chilli,
finely chopped

1 garlic clove, crushed

juice of 1 lime

To serve:

Gaz's "Guac" (see page 86)

gluten-free buns

gluten-free nachos

Preheat the oven to 180°C
(350°F) and line a baking tray with
greaseproof paper.

To make the burgers, simply add all
the ingredients to a blender. Pulse
until the mixture starts to combine.
You may have to scrape down the
sides of the blender a couple of
times but don't over-blend the mix
or it will turn into a paste. Keep
some texture in those burgers!

Once blended, form the mixture
into 4 burger patties with your
hands. I find it easier to divide it
into 4 evenly sized balls, then press
and shape them into a burger
shape on the work surface. Place
the burgers onto the baking tray.

Preheat a non-stick frying pan
over a medium heat and add a
little coconut oil. Fry the burgers,
a couple at a time, until golden

on each side (for approximately
2 minutes per side). Place the
burgers back on the tray, then
straight into the oven to cook
through for 12 minutes.

Meanwhile, prepare the tomato
salsa (mix all the ingredients
together in a bowl) and the
burger garnishes.

Once the burgers are out of the
oven, stack up your Mexican
burger. First spread a layer of Gaz's
guac, then put the burger on top,
followed by a dollop of salsa and
some nacho crisps.

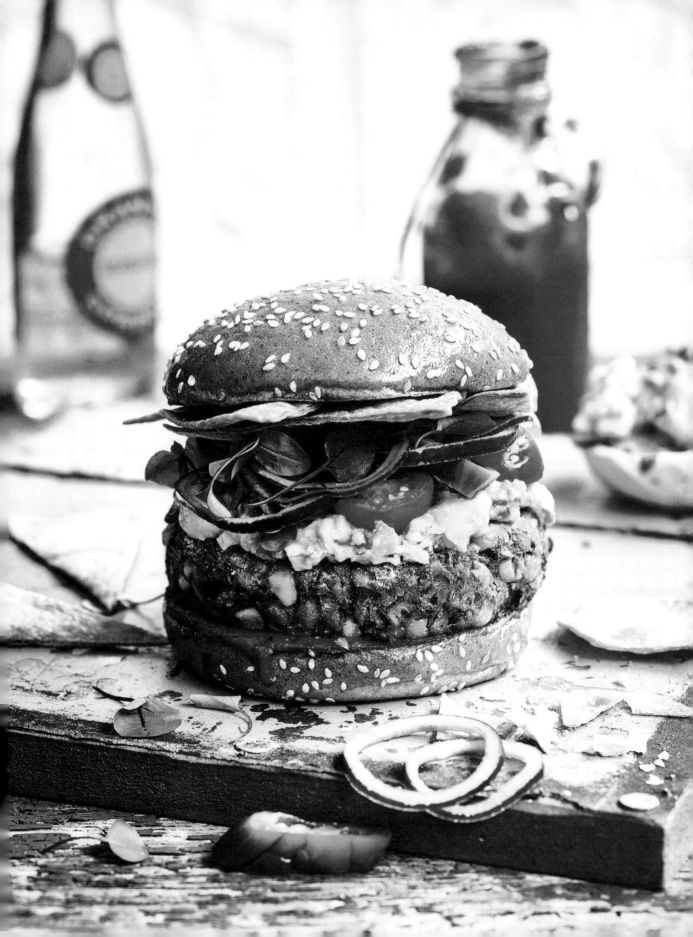

THE MAINS

Sriracha "Meatballs" with Noodles & Grilled Vegetables

Beetroot Risotto with Candied Walnuts & Beetroot Crisps

"Mac & Cheese" with Coconut "Bacon" Bits

Baked Chickpea-Crumbed Aubergine, Courgette & Red Pepper Katsu Curry

"Fish" & Chips with Tartare Sauce & Mushy Minted Peas

Epic Raw Lasagne

Smoked Pea & Chickpea Pizza

Seitan Fillet "Steak" Wellington

Ultimate Vegan Roast

Coconut Stew, Rice & Peas with Fried Plantain

SRIRACHA "MEATBALLS" WITH NOODLES & GRILLED VEGETABLES

These punchy little "meatballs" are so delicious. Sriracha is one of my all-time favourite sauces – the spicy tanginess it adds to this dish is just perfect. Make sure you get some nice charring on the grilled vegetables as it adds lots of flavour.

SERVES 4

For the meatballs:

1 x 300-g (10-oz) firm block of tofu, water drained and excess water removed

3 spring onions (scallions), very finely sliced

3 garlic cloves, crushed

1 small red chilli, finely chopped

handful of coriander (cilantro), chopped

1 tbsp Egg Replacement (see page 32)

4 tbsp buckwheat flour

2 tbsp sesame oil

1 tbsp tomato puree

3 tbsp Sriracha sauce

1 tbsp coconut oil, for sautéing

For the sauce:

5 tbsp Sriracha sauce

5 tbsp tomato ketchup

3 tbsp maple syrup

5 tbsp water

To serve:

300g (10½oz) rice noodles

vegetables (such as asparagus, pak choi, Tenderstem broccoli, radishes, carrots, sugarsnap peas)

cucumber ribbons

mixed sesame seeds

fresh coriander (cilantro)

Preheat the oven to 180°C (350°F) and line a baking tray with greaseproof paper.

First up, make those meatballs. Mash the tofu with a potato masher in a large mixing bowl, until it's broken up into small pieces. Add all the other meatball ingredients to the bowl and stir until well incorporated. If the mix is still slightly wet, add a couple of extra tbsp flour.

Now it's time to form the mixture into balls. Take 1 large tablespoon of mixture and form into a ball with your hands. Repeat until you've used up all the mixture. Lightly flour your hands between each meatball to stop the mixture from sticking. Place the meatballs onto the lined baking tray as you go.

Cook the rice noodles according to the packet instructions and prepare your vegetables for grilling.

Heat a non-stick frying pan over a low heat, add the coconut oil and sauté the meatballs in small quantities, until golden. This should take approximately 3 minutes per batch. Place them back onto the tray, then into the oven to cook through for 10 minutes.

While the meatballs are in the oven, mix together the sauce ingredients in a small saucepan and heat gently until you're ready to serve. Grill your vegetables on a hot griddle pan until charred.

Once the meatballs are cooked, serve in a large bowl with the rice noodles, lots of the grilled vegetables, the cucumber ribbons and plenty of sauce.

Sprinkle over mixed sesame seeds and chopped coriander just before serving.

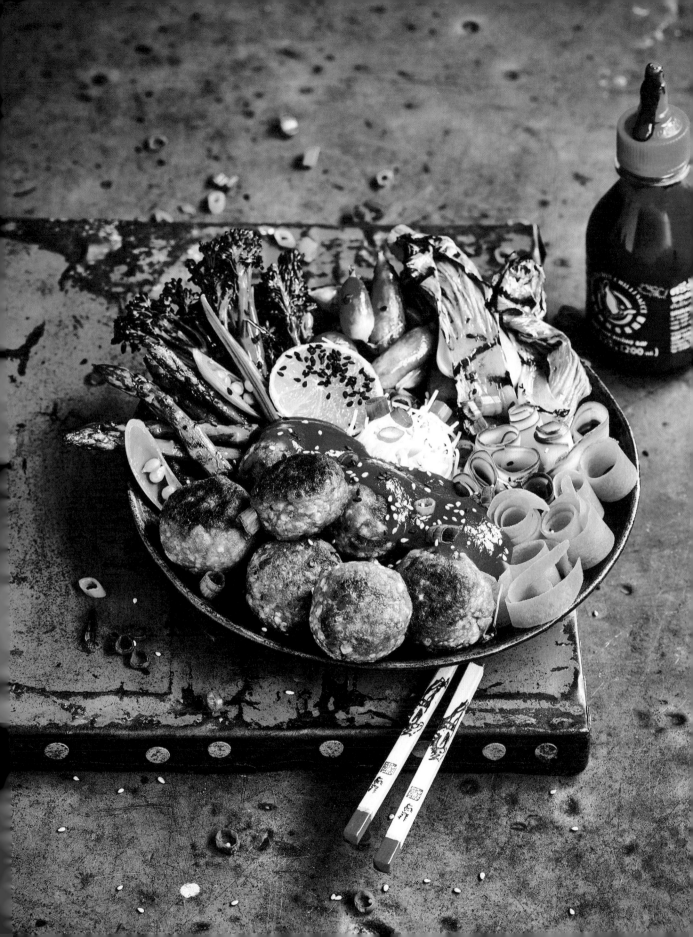

BEETROOT RISOTTO WITH CANDIED WALNUTS & BEETROOT CRISPS

Super-purple in colour, this risotto certainly has loads of vibrancy! The crunchy, caramelized walnuts are a perfect match for the thyme-flavoured beetroot risotto, and the crispy beetroot adds an extra dimension of taste and texture.

SERVES 4

3 raw beetroots (beets), peeled

3 tbsp olive oil

4 shallots, finely chopped

2 garlic cloves, minced

2 sprigs fresh thyme, leaves picked

200g (2 cups) risotto (Arborio) rice

240ml (1 cup) vegan white wine

1 litre (4 cups) hot Vegetable Stock (see page 31), plus a little extra

2 tbsp nutritional yeast

sea salt and pepper

For the beetroot crisps:

1 raw beetroot (beet), peeled

1 tbsp olive oil

sea salt and pepper

For the candied walnuts:

250g ($\frac{1}{4}$ cup) unrefined caster (granulated) sugar

1 tbsp vegan "butter"

100g (1 cup) walnuts

To serve:

fresh rocket (arugula)

Preheat the oven to 180°C (350°F) and line 3 baking trays with greaseproof paper.

First up, chop the 3 beetroots into cubes, then spread out on one of the baking trays. Drizzle with 2 tbsp of the olive oil and sprinkle over some seasoning, then bake in the oven for 45 minutes, or until soft.

Now make the beetroot crisps: using a mandoline on its thinnest setting, slice the beetroot into a bowl. Add the olive oil and a pinch of seasoning. Give it a good old mix until each piece is covered, then lay each piece onto another lined baking tray, making sure they don't overlap. Transfer to the oven on a shelf below the other beetroot to crisp up – around 15 minutes but check them every 5 minutes.

For the candied walnuts, heat the sugar and the butter in a non-stick, heavy-based saucepan over a medium heat. Once the sugar and butter have turned into a golden caramel, carefully add the walnuts. Give them a light stir so each walnut has a good coating, then remove from the pan and transfer to the last lined baking tray, making sure they are separated. Leave to set for 5 minutes. (They will keep in a cool, dry place for up to 3 days.)

When the beetroot is nearly done, start making your risotto. Sauté the shallots, garlic and fresh thyme in the rest of the olive oil, in a large saucepan over a medium heat. Stir often and make sure they don't catch or burn; just let them soften.

Once the shallots are soft, reduce the heat and add all of the risotto rice. Stir well for around 1 minute, making sure the rice is coated.

Add the white wine and stir every now and then until it has all been absorbed by the rice. Now start adding around a cup of stock at a time, stirring until it's absorbed, until you have used up all the stock – this will take about 20 minutes, after which the rice should almost look creamy. If not, add more stock.

Check the rice is cooked. If it isn't, add a splash more stock, and carry on cooking for a few minutes. Once the rice is soft enough to eat, gently stir in the roasted beetroot cubes and the nutritional yeast. Check for seasoning and add a pinch of sea salt and pepper if necessary.

To serve, add generous spoonfuls of the risotto. Then top with the candied walnuts, beetroot crisps and fresh rocket.

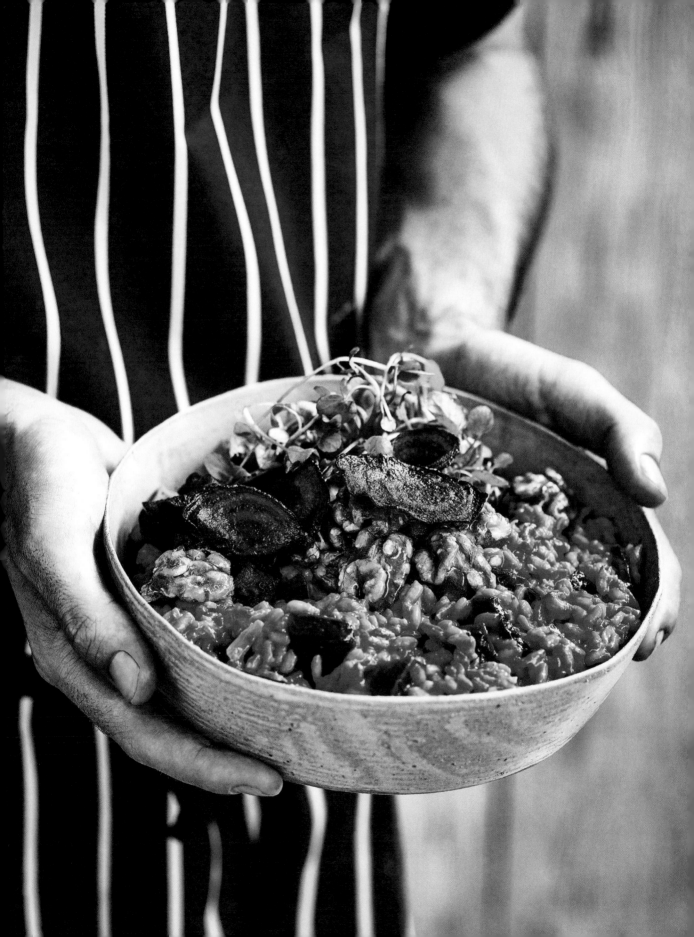

"MAC & CHEESE" WITH COCONUT "BACON" BITS

A classic that I had to veganize, this is so creamy and moreish, you won't believe it. The coconut bits are smoky and have an incredible maple "bacon" flavour. They also add a great texture.

SERVES 4

250g (2 cups) macaroni (or gluten-free pasta)

1 tbsp olive oil

½ head of cauliflower, cut into small florets

1 small onion, finely chopped

2 garlic cloves, crushed

1 leek, washed and finely chopped

50g (½ cup) almonds

300ml (2½ cups) almond Milk (see page 12)

1 tbsp English mustard

1 tsp paprika

1 tbsp fresh thyme leaves

1 x 400-ml (14-oz) can coconut milk

5 tbsp nutritional yeast

salt and pepper

For the coconut "bacon":

80g (1 cup) coconut flakes

2 tbsp maple syrup

2 tbsp liquid smoke

2 tbsp soy sauce

1 tbsp coconut oil

Preheat the oven to 180°C (350°F) and line a baking tray with greaseproof paper.

First make the coconut bacon: stir all the ingredients together in a mixing bowl. Once all the coconut flakes are well coated, spread out over the lined baking tray. Bake in the oven for 10–15 minutes until golden and crisp. Check the coconut a couple of times and give it a stir during cooking as it can easily burn.

Bring a large pan of salted water to the boil and cook the macaroni for 8–10 minutes, until al dente.

Blanch the cauliflower florets in boiling water for 3 minutes, then drain.

Meanwhile, in a large saucepan, add a small amount of oil before sautéing the onion, garlic, leek and blanched cauliflower. Cook over a low heat, stirring often.

Blend the almonds and almond milk until smooth, then add to the pan containing the onion mixture to make a sauce.

Drain the pasta and set aside.

Add the mustard, paprika and thyme to the sauce, giving it a stir before adding the cooked pasta.

Add the coconut milk, yeast and a pinch of salt and pepper before cooking for a further 1–2 minutes over a low heat, until it is thick and creamy.

Serve immediately, garnishing with a pinch of paprika and the crispy coconut bacon bits.

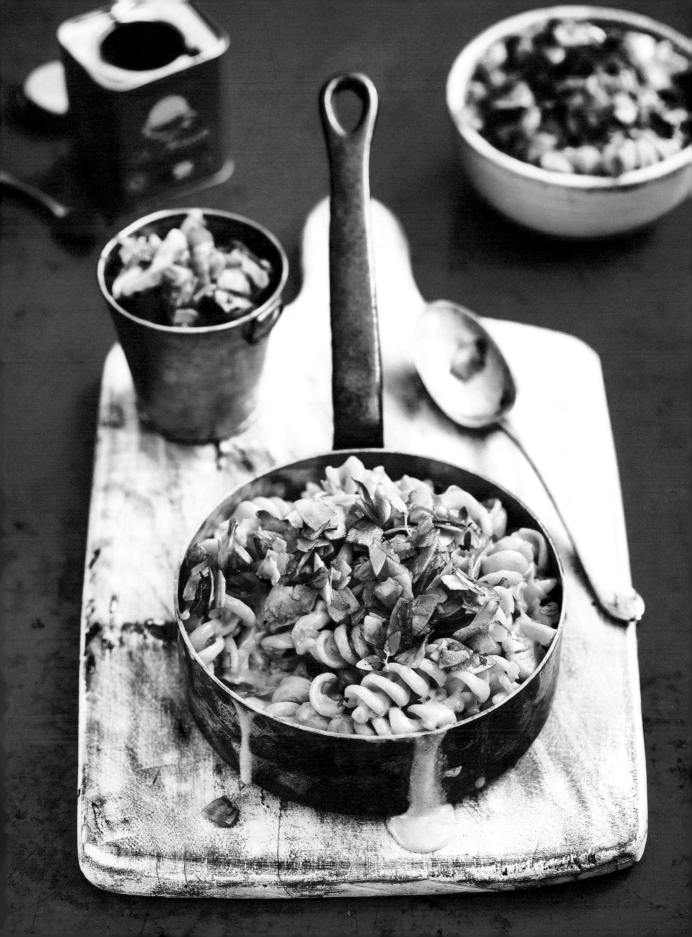

BAKED CHICKPEA-CRUMBED AUBERGINE, COURGETTE & RED PEPPER KATSU CURRY

One of my favourite meals to make, this version is made a lot healthier by coating the aubergine, courgette and red pepper in gluten-free breadcrumbs, then baking them. The mix of textures makes this dish a delight to eat – I love Japanese flavours!

SERVES 4

4 tbsp cornflour (cornstarch)

4 tbsp gluten-free flour

60g (1 cup) chickpea crumbs or gluten-free breadcrumbs

½ aubergine (eggplant), cut into 2.5-cm (1-inch) cubes

½ courgette (zucchini), cut into 2.5-cm (1-inch) cubes

1 red (bell) pepper, cut into 2.5-cm (1-inch) cubes

2 tbsp sesame oil

pinch sea salt and pepper

For the Katsu curry sauce:

1 tbsp coconut oil

1 red onion, finely chopped

1 garlic clove, crushed

½ banana, finely chopped

1 carrot, finely chopped

1 tbsp curry powder

1 tsp garam masala

½ tsp chilli powder

350ml (1½ cups) Vegetable Stock (see page 31)

2 tbsp soy sauce

1 tbsp tomato puree

To serve:

sushi rice

watercress

pickled onion and radish (see page 92)

mixed sesame seeds

Preheat the oven to 180°C (350°F) and line a baking tray with greaseproof paper.

Mix the cornflour in a bowl with enough water to make a thick, sticky paste. Put the flour in a shallow bowl and the chickpea crumbs in another.

Individually, dip the vegetable pieces into the flour, then the cornflour paste (making sure they are well covered), then coat in the chickpea crumbs. Place the coated vegetables onto the lined baking tray as you go.

Lightly drizzle over the sesame oil and sprinkle over the seasoning, then bake in the oven for about 25 minutes.

Meanwhile, make the Katsu sauce. Add the coconut oil to a small saucepan and melt over a low heat. Add the onion, garlic, banana and carrot, and sweat for a couple minutes until soft. Add the spices and cook for a further couple minutes, stirring often.

Next add the stock, soy sauce and tomato puree, and simmer over a low heat for 10 minutes to thicken slightly. Use a hand stick blender to blend the sauce lightly until smooth.

Once the coated vegetables are crispy and golden, remove them from the oven until you're ready to serve.

Serve the crispy vegetables with sushi rice and generous amounts of the sauce poured over. Add a little watercress and pickled onion and radish on the side and finish with a sprinkle of mixed sesame seeds.

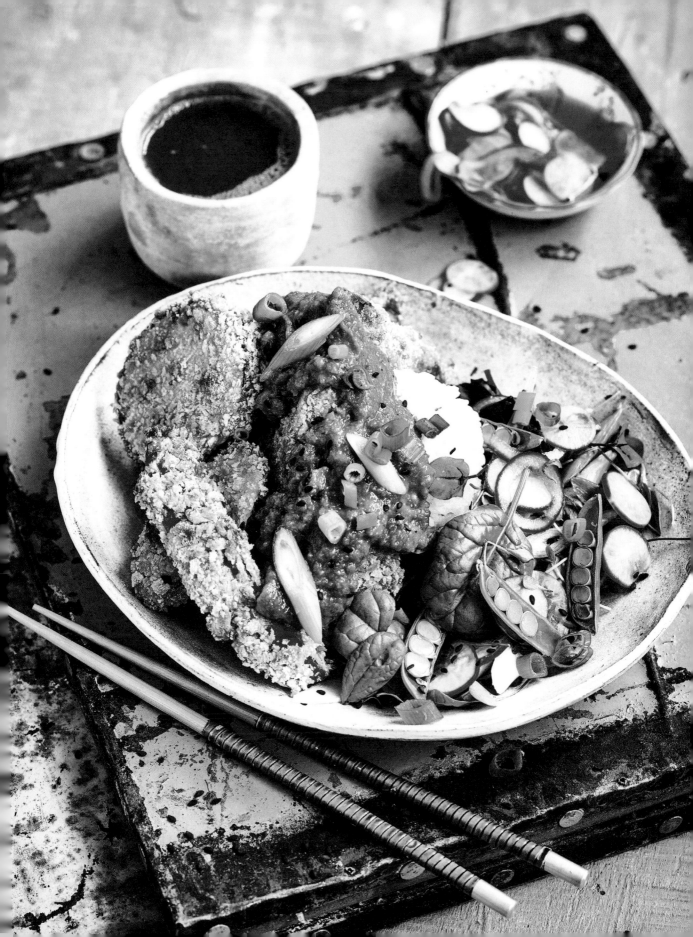

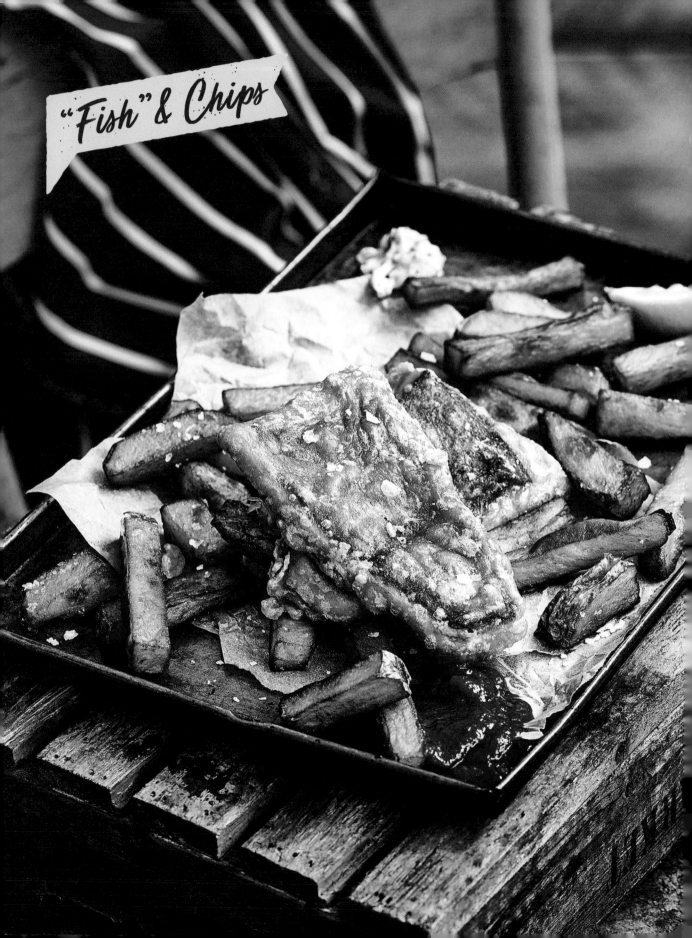

"Fish" & Chips

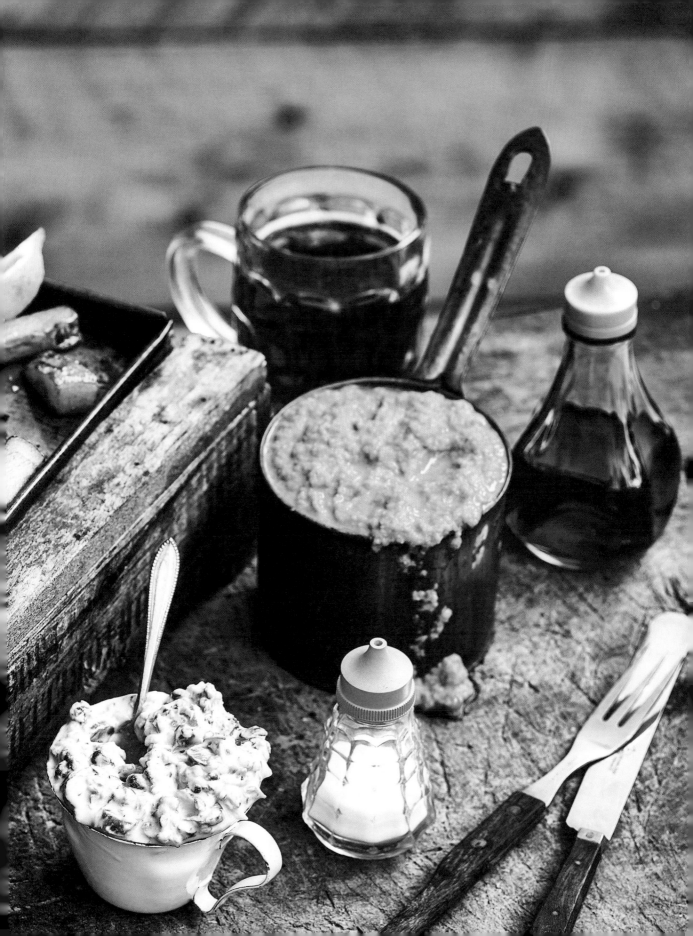

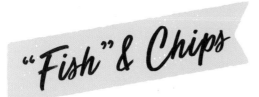

WITH TARTARE SAUCE & MUSHY MINTED PEAS

When my "veganized" version of this British classic went viral on
YouTube, lots of people found my channel from this video!
It's a great treat and will fool any of your non-vegan friends.

SERVES 4–5

For the chips:

5 medium Maris Piper potatoes

2 tbsp plain (all-purpose) flour

4 tbsp olive oil

pinch sea salt and pepper

For the "fish":

approximately 1 litre
(4 cups) sunflower oil

1 x 400-g (14-oz) firm
block of tofu, drained and
excess water removed

1 large (20 x 18-cm/8 x
7-inch) sheet of nori

juice of 1 lemon

50g (¹⁄₄ cup) plain
(all-purpose) flour

50g (¹⁄₄ cup) cornflour (cornstarch)

75ml (¹⁄₃ cup) vegan beer

75ml (¹⁄₃ cup) soda water

pinch sea salt

For the mushy minted peas:

olive oil, for frying

2 shallots, finely chopped

300g (2 cups) frozen peas

235ml (1 cup) Vegetable
Stock (see page 31)

2 tbsp fresh lemon juice

1 tbsp finely chopped fresh mint

pinch salt and pepper

For the tartare sauce:

250g (1 cup) "Mayonnaise"
(see page 24)

3 tbsp capers, drained
and roughly chopped

3 tbsp roughly chopped gherkins

1 small shallot, finely chopped

1 tbsp fresh lemon juice

3 tbsp chopped fresh parsley

pinch sea salt and pepper

Preheat the oven to 180°C (350°F) and line a large baking tray with greaseproof paper.

First prepare your chips: wash and slice the potatoes into chip shapes of your choice. I like chunky chips and I also leave the skin on but it's up to you if you want to peel them or not.

Cover the chips with water in a large saucepan, add a pinch of salt, then place over a medium heat. Bring to the boil, boil for 2 minutes, then drain. Par-boiling the chips helps create a super-soft inside – I highly recommend doing this if you like your chips chunky.

Spread the par-boiled chips on the baking tray and sprinkle with the plain flour, making sure each chip is lightly covered. Drizzle over the olive oil and season with salt and pepper, then bake for around 25–30 minutes, or until golden and crispy.

While your chips are cooking, it's time to make the "fish" element. Pour the sunflower oil into a large saucepan set over a medium heat, or a deep-fat fryer set to 180°C (350°F). If using a saucepan, only half fill it to prevent it overflowing when you put the tofu in.

Cut the tofu block into rectangles or fillet shapes. Using scissors, cut the nori sheet into pieces the same shape and size as the tofu fillets. The nori resembles fish skin and also has a great taste-of-the-sea flavour.

Lay the nori onto the tofu and squeeze over some of the lemon juice to help it stick. Set aside while you quickly whisk up your beer batter.

Combine the flours and salt in a mixing bowl, then pour in the beer and water. Mix together with a wooden spoon until it forms a thick batter. Set aside to rest for a few minutes.

Meanwhile, make the mushy minted peas. Sauté the shallots in a saucepan with a little olive oil, until soft. Add the peas, stock and lemon juice, and cook over a medium heat until piping hot. Use a hand stick blender to blitz until mushy, then stir in the mint and a pinch of seasoning. Keep warm until ready to serve.

Combine all the ingredients for the tartare sauce in a mixing bowl, then set aside until ready to serve.

At this point your oil should be hot enough to cook the tofu. You should be able to see a light haze coming off the top of the oil in the saucepan but, to be sure, drop a cube of bread into the oil – if it floats to the top quickly and turns golden, your oil is hot enough.

Dip each piece of nori-lined tofu into the batter individually and then lower into the oil very carefully. Cook until the batter is golden, for approximately 4 minutes, then transfer to a plate lined with kitchen paper to drain off excess oil. Sprinkle with salt.

Remove the chips from the oven, serve with the tofu fish, mushy peas and tartare sauce.

EPIC RAW LASAGNE

**This lasagne is delightfully light, nutritious and refreshing.
For a raw meal, it's also very substantial and has an incredible blend of flavours.**

SERVES 4

For the "cheese" sauce:

150g (1 cup) raw cashew nuts

2 tbsp fresh lemon juice

2 tbsp nutritional yeast

1 tsp fresh thyme

180ml ($^3/_4$ cup) almond
Milk (see page 12)

pinch sea salt and pepper

For the rich tomato sauce:

45g ($^1/_3$ cup) sun-dried
tomatoes in oil

1 beefsteak tomato

$^1/_2$ garlic clove

2 tbsp smoked olive oil

4 tbsp filtered water

1 tbsp fresh lemon juice

1 tbsp fresh chopped basil

For the herby pesto:

handful of fresh basil

handful of fresh parsley

$^1/_2$ ripe avocado

2 tbsp extra virgin olive oil

60ml ($^1/_4$ cup) filtered water

80g ($^1/_2$ cup) pine nuts

1 garlic clove

2 tbsp lemon juice

pinch sea salt and pepper

For the vegetable layers:

2 courgettes (zucchinis)

8 radishes

2 beefsteak tomatoes

handful of fresh spinach

handful of fresh basil leaves

Soak the cashew nuts in water for at least 1 hour.

Make the tomato sauce: drain away the soaking water from the sun-dried tomatoes then put them in a blender with the rest of the ingredients. Pulse until just combined (I like my tomato sauce to have a bit of texture to it). Pour the sauce into a bowl, cover with cling film (plastic wrap) and chill in the fridge until ready to assemble the lasagne. Wash the blender.

Now make the "cheese" sauce: drain the soaking water from the cashews. Blitz the nuts with the rest of the ingredients, until you have a silky smooth sauce. Scrape the sauce into a bowl, cover with cling film and chill in the fridge until ready to assemble the lasagne. Wash the blender.

Next the herby pesto: it's the same process. Simply blitz all the ingredients until smooth. Add a touch more olive oil or some water if your pesto isn't wet enough.

Now prepare the vegetables: using a mandoline on its finest setting, carefully slice the courgettes lengthways into long strips. (Make sure you use the mandoline guard.) Slicing the courgettes super finely means that you don't have to marinate them in anything, which would spoil their nutrients.

Use a sharp knife to slice the radishes and tomatoes as finely as you can. Wash the spinach and basil leaves.

To assemble the lasagne, you can use a square or ring or just layer everything up in a tray. First make a layer of courgette slices, followed by slices of radishes, tomatoes, spinach, a layer of tomato sauce, then cheese sauce, then pesto. Repeat the stacking until you have a little bit of everything in. Then remove the ring, if using, and drizzle some sauce down the side.

Garnish with a sprinkle of cracked black pepper and a few fresh basil leaves on top.

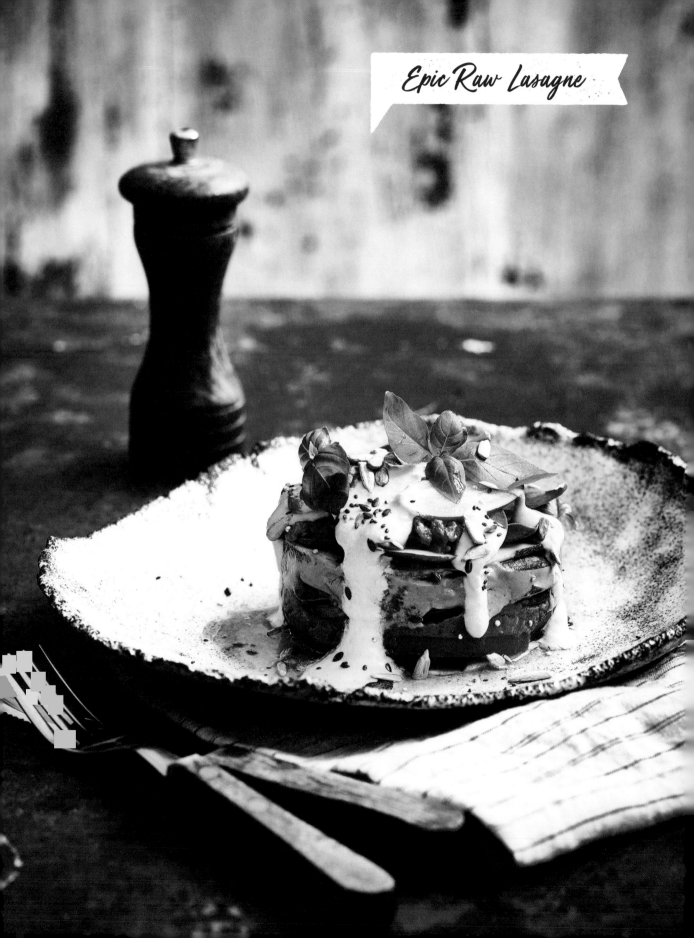

Epic Raw Lasagne

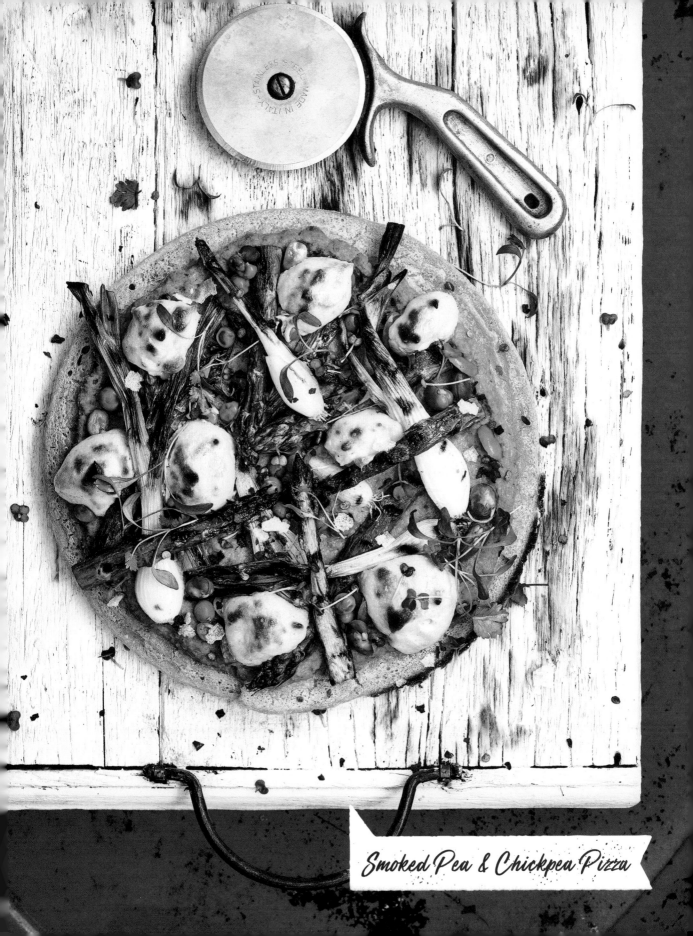

Smoked Pea & Chickpea Pizza

SMOKED PEA & CHICKPEA PIZZA

This is a healthier alternative to pizza – it's big on flavour and very colourful. Chargrilling the asparagus and spring onions adds a whole new dimension to the flavour. This chickpea flatbread hails from Italy, where it is also known as "socca".

MAKES 2 x 25-cm (10-inch) PIZZAS

For the chickpea flatbread:

135g (1½ cups) chickpea (gram) flour

pinch salt and pepper

352ml (1½ cups) water

1 tbsp olive oil

For the smoked peas:

3 shallots, finely chopped

olive oil, for frying

195g (1½ cups) frozen peas

60ml (¼ cup) hot Vegetable Stock (see page 31)

1 tbsp fresh lemon juice

½ tsp liquid smoke (or ½ tsp smoked paprika)

pinch salt and pepper

Toppings:

8 asparagus tips, trimmed and washed

8 spring onions (scallions), topped and tailed, and washed

80g (½ cup) frozen broad beans, defrosted and skinned

zest of ½ lemon

3 tbsp "Cream Cheese" (see page 15

To garnish:

pea shoots

fresh mint leaves

First make the chickpea flatbread batter: put the flour and seasoning into a mixing bowl. Grab yourself a whisk, then whisk in the water and olive oil. The mixture should have a thick batter-like consistency. Cover the bowl with cling film (plastic wrap) and pop the batter into the fridge to rest for 20 minutes. This gives you time to prepare the rest of the pizza components.

To make the smoked peas, sauté the shallots in a little olive oil in a small saucepan over a medium heat, until soft. Add the peas, stock and lemon juice, and heat through, until the peas are piping hot. Using a hand stick blender, blend until almost smooth. I like a little bit of texture, so I don't blitz it all the way. Add a couple drops of liquid smoke or smoked paprika, stir to combine and set the pea puree aside until needed.

Heat a griddle pan until smoking hot, then add a little olive oil. (Make sure your extractor fan is on for this!) Grill the asparagus and spring onions quickly until lightly charred, then remove from the heat and set aside. Make sure the pan is really hot – you just want to char the outside of the asparagus, not cook it.

Preheat the grill (broiler) and heat a 28-cm (11-inch) ovenproof, non-stick frying pan over a low heat. Add a little olive oil, ladle in all of the chickpea batter and cook for 2 minutes. Carefully transfer the pan and place under the grill for 2 minutes. (This saves you having to flip it over in the pan!)

After 2 minutes, carefully remove the pan from the grill; the flatbread should be nice and golden.

Spoon over the smoked pea mixture, then top with the grilled spring onions and asparagus. Sprinkle over the broad beans and lemon zest and add a few dollops of cashew cheese.

Place the topped pizza back under the grill to cook for a further 2 minutes.

Serve with a sprinkling of pea shoots and fresh mint leaves.

SEITAN FILLET "STEAK" WELLINGTON

Serve this on a special occasion with the Mixed Lemon Greens (see page 162) and your guests will be so impressed. It has all the flavours of a traditional beef Wellington. If you didn't want to make a seitan "steak" filling you can always replace it with sautéed portobello mushrooms.

SERVES 8–10

500g (17½oz) Rough Puff Pastry (see page 30), or shop-bought vegan puff pastry

2 tbsp almond Milk (see page 12)

1 tbsp extra virgin olive oil

2 tsp agave nectar

pinch sea salt

For the fillet "steak" – wet:

160ml (⅔ cup) hot Vegetable Stock (see page 31)

10g (½ cup) dried porcini mushrooms

olive oil, for frying

1 red onion, finely chopped

2 garlic cloves, finely chopped

120ml (½ cup) red wine

50g (¼ cup) chopped cooked beetroot (beet)

50g (½ cup) canned black beans

3 tbsp tomato puree

1 tbsp soy sauce

1 tbsp balsamic vinegar

1 tbsp brown rice miso paste

1 tsp Marmite

1 tsp dried sage

1 tsp dried oregano

¼ tsp ground cloves

1 tsp cayenne pepper

½ tsp dried rosemary

1 tsp dried tarragon

1 tsp sea salt

1 tbsp cracked black pepper

For the fillet "steak" – dry :

300g (2¾ cups) seitan (vital wheat gluten)

50g (½ cup) chickpea (gram) flour

2 tbsp nutritional yeast

For the broth:

1 litre (4 cups) Vegetable Stock (see page 31)

240ml (1 cup) red wine

1 tbsp miso paste

1 onion, peeled and quartered

3 garlic cloves

2 cloves

1 bay leaf

2 sprigs rosemary

3 tbsp dried porcini mushrooms

Optional herbs and spices for steak:

¼ tsp dried sage

¼ tsp dried oregano

¼ tsp cayenne pepper

¼ tsp dried rosemary

¼ tsp dried tarragon

1 tbsp cracked black pepper

For the filling:

450g (6 cups) mixed mushrooms

2 garlic cloves, crushed

1 tbsp fresh rosemary leaves, finely chopped

handful of spinach, wilted

2 tbsp English mustard

[Continued on page 140...]

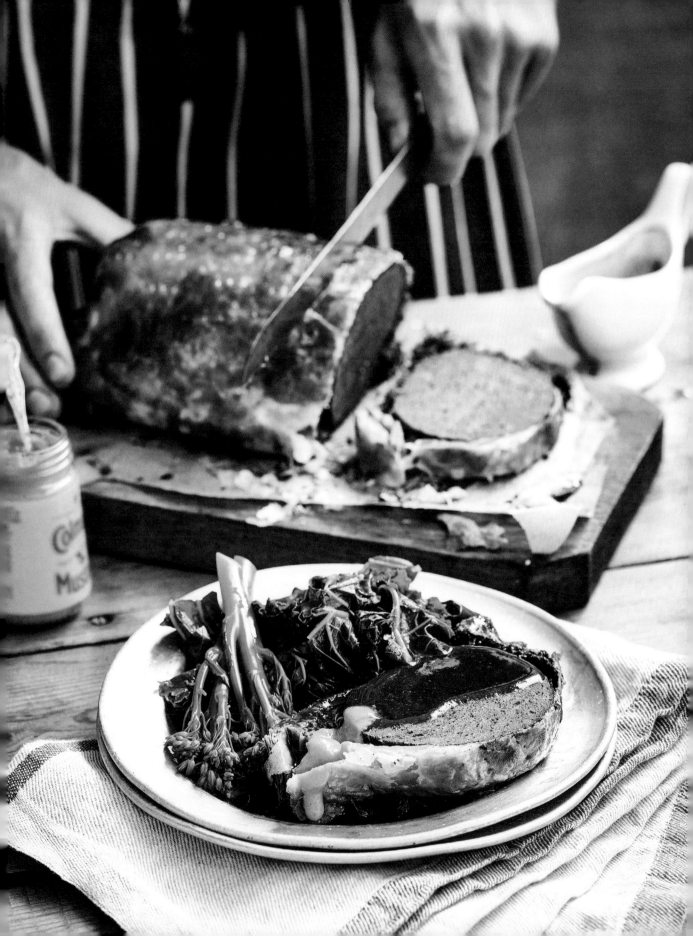

SEITAN FILLET "STEAK" WELLINGTON (CONT.)

For the wet ingredients: mix the hot vegetable stock with the porcini and set aside for 5 minutes for the porcini to rehydrate.

Heat a non-stick saucepan and add a touch of olive oil. When the pan is hot, add the onion and garlic, reduce the heat and allow them to soften and lightly caramelize for around 2 minutes, stirring often.

Remove the pan from the heat and tip the onions and garlic into a blender together with the remaining wet ingredients, plus the mushrooms and stock. Let the mixture sit for 5 minutes to cool before you blitz. This gives you time to prep the dry ingredients.

Combine the wheat gluten, chickpea flour and nutritional yeast in a large mixing bowl.

Blitz the wet mixture until smooth, then pour into the mixing bowl of dry ingredients and quickly stir with a spatula until everything is well combined into a "dough".

Use your hands to knead the dough for 10 minutes in the bowl or on a clean work surface. It may be quite wet so sprinkle some chickpea flour on the surface. The tougher you are when kneading, the more of a bite/meat-like texture your seitan will have when cooked, so be firm!

After kneading, return the dough to the bowl and cover with a clean tea towel to rest and firm up for 15 minutes.

While the dough is resting, heat all the broth ingredients in a large saucepan and bring it all to the boil, then reduce to simmering.

Shape the dough into a rough fillet shape to make it easier for wrapping in pastry. Sprinkle the fillet with the optional herbs and spices if using. Lightly wrap the fillet in muslin/cheesecloth and tie the ends – this just holds the shape.

Lower the fillet into the lightly simmering broth, pop the lid on and cook for 1 hour and 15 minutes, or until firm to touch. Make sure the broth is only ever just simmering, never boiling. I carefully turn the seitan fillet over a couple of times to make sure it cooks evenly.

Meanwhile, make the mushroom filling. Blitz the mushrooms, garlic and rosemary in a blender. Heat a non-stick frying pan, add the mushroom mixture and cook until all the natural water has come out of the mushrooms. Lightly season with salt and pepper. Spoon into a bowl, cover with cling film (plastic wrap) and chill in the fridge until completely cool.

Once the fillet has simmered in the broth for 75 minutes, check it's firm.

If so, remove it from the broth and place onto a plate. If not, simmer for a few more minutes. Allow to cool to room temperature. Don't discard the broth – reduce it down to create the most flavoursome gravy to go with the Wellington once it's cooked.

Preheat the oven to 190°C (375°F) and line a baking tray with greaseproof paper.

Mix the almond milk, extra virgin olive oil, agave nectar and salt together in a bowl to use as a glaze.

Roll out the pastry into a rectangle around 3mm (1/8 inch) thick, and 25 x 36cm (10 x 14 inches). Spread the chilled mushroom mixture onto the pastry, leaving a 2.5-cm (1-inch) border around the edge. Top the mushrooms with a layer of the wilted spinach. Lightly brush the fillet with the mustard, then place the fillet lengthways towards the bottom of the pastry on top of the mushroom and spinach. Brush the border with the milk glaze.

Roll the pastry over the fillet so that the join is underneath. Seal the edges, brush the glaze all over, then transfer onto the baking tray.

Bake for 25 minutes, or until the pastry is crisp and golden. Serve with the reduced-broth gravy.

ULTIMATE VEGAN ROAST

This nut roast is far from boring and is full of incredible flavours and excellent nutrients. It is perfect for special occasions or a Sunday lunch, served with gravy and Mixed Lemon Greens (see page 162).

SERVES 8–10

3 tbsp extra virgin olive oil

1 red onion, finely chopped

2 garlic cloves

1 red (bell) pepper, cubed

1 leek, washed and finely chopped

200g (1 cup) peeled and diced butternut squash

75g (1 cup) roughly chopped chestnut mushrooms

60g ($\frac{1}{2}$ cup) roughly chopped vacuum-packed chestnuts

$\frac{1}{2}$ tsp paprika

$\frac{1}{2}$ tsp cayenne pepper

$\frac{1}{4}$ tsp ground cinnamon

1 sprig fresh rosemary, leaves finely chopped

10 fresh sage leaves, finely chopped

sea salt and pepper

zest of 1 lemon

75g (1 cup) mixed nuts

75g (1 cup) red lentils, cooked

45g ($\frac{1}{2}$ cup) gluten-free breadcrumbs

50g ($\frac{1}{4}$ cup) dried cranberries, roughly chopped

50g ($\frac{1}{4}$ cup) dried apricots, roughly chopped

50g ($\frac{1}{4}$ cup) sun-dried tomatoes, roughly chopped

4 tbsp Egg Replacement (see page 32)

Preheat the oven to 180°C (350°F) and grease and line a 900-g (2-lb) loaf tin with baking paper.

Heat the olive oil in a large saucepan over a medium heat, add the onion, garlic, pepper, leek, squash, mushrooms and chestnuts, and sauté for 2 minutes, stirring often. Add the spices, herbs, some seasoning and the lemon zest, and stir to combine.

Reduce the heat and cook for 8–10 minutes more, stirring every now and then. You just want all the flavours to marry together and the vegetables to slightly soften.

While the vegetables are cooking, blitz the nuts in the blender until they are a crumb-like consistency, then tip into a large mixing bowl.

Add the lentils, breadcrumbs, dried cranberries and apricots, and sun-dried tomatoes.

Once the vegetables have softened, add to the bowl, mix everything together with a wooden spoon, then add the egg replacer and stir to combine. This helps everything bind together.

Scrape the mixture into your lined tin and press it down as much as you can. Cover with foil, then transfer to the oven to roast for 35–40 minutes. Once cooked, let it cool for 5 minutes before turning it out of the tin onto a serving plate. Slice into 4-cm (1$\frac{1}{2}$-inch) pieces.

COCONUT STEW, RICE & PEAS WITH FRIED PLANTAIN

Get those Caribbean flavours going with this beautiful, creamy coconut stew served here with my all-time favourite ingredient, plantain. When it's fried in coconut oil it caramelizes so beautifully.

SERVES 5

1 tbsp coconut oil

2 red onion, cut into chunks

3-cm (1¼-inch) piece of fresh ginger, finely chopped

2 garlic cloves, crushed

1 red chilli, deseeded and finely chopped

3 tsp jerk seasoning

pinch sea salt and pepper

1 medium butternut squash, peeled and cubed

2 Maris Piper potatoes, peeled and cubed

1 medium aubergine (eggplant), cubed

1 courgette (zucchini), cubed

1 red (bell) pepper, cubed

1 x 400-ml (14-oz) can coconut milk

295ml (1½ cups) Vegetable Stock (see page 31)

2 tbsp tomato puree

juice of ½ lime

165g (1 cup) canned chickpeas, drained and rinsed

75g (½ cup) toasted cashew nuts

handful of spinach

100g (1 cup) peeled and cubed mango

For the rice and peas:

1 x 400-g (14-oz) can kidney beans, liquid reserved

1 x 400-ml (14-oz) can coconut milk

400ml (1²/₃ cups) Vegetable Stock (see page 31)

3 tbsp fresh thyme leaves

pinch sea salt and black pepper

450g (2 cups) long grain rice, rinsed

For the fried plantain:

2 medium plantains, peeled and cut into 1-cm (½-in) discs

2 tbsp coconut oil

First make the curry: heat a large, lidded saucepan over a low heat and add the coconut oil. Once the pan is hot, add the onion, ginger, garlic and chilli. Sweat for a couple of minutes while stirring. Add the jerk seasoning and a pinch of salt and pepper, and cook for 2 minutes more.

Now add the squash, potatoes, aubergine, courgette and pepper, and sauté for 4–5 minutes until the vegetables have softened slightly.

Pour in the coconut milk, stock, tomato puree and lime. Pop the lid

on and simmer for 15–20 minutes, stirring every now and then.

While the stew is cooking, prepare the rice and peas. Pour the contents of the can of beans into a medium saucepan with the coconut milk and stock. Add the thyme and seasoning. Bring to the boil, then stir in the rice. Allow to boil for a couple of minutes before popping the lid on, turning the heat down and leaving it to simmer for 15 minutes, or until the rice has absorbed all the liquid and is fluffy.

After the stew has simmered for 15 minutes, check the squash and potatoes are cooked. If not, continue to cook for a few more minutes. When they are cooked, stir in the chickpeas, toasted cashews, spinach and mango.

Simmer for 3 more minutes then turn off the heat.

Just before you're ready to serve, fry the plantain. Melt the coconut oil in a large, non-stick frying pan over a medium heat. Fry the plantain slices on both sides, until they're caramelized and golden.

Serve plenty of rice and peas, stew and plantain in large bowls, with a wedge of lime and fresh coriander sprinkled on top.

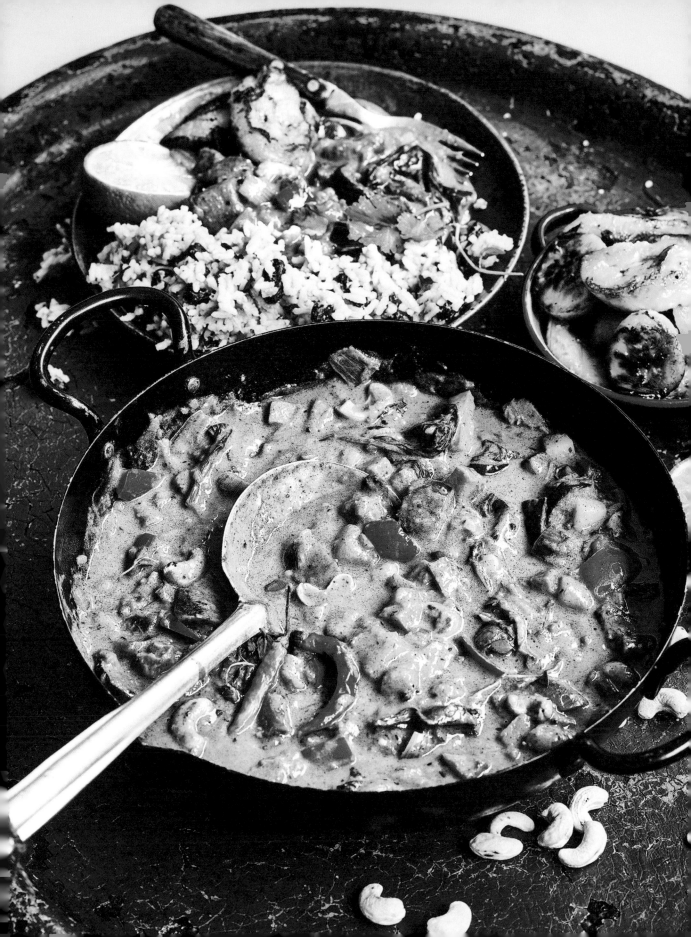

SALADS

Nutty Wild Rice Salad

Asparagus & Kale
Caesar Salad

Beetroot, Sweet Potato,
Orange & Walnut Salad

Raw Root Salad with Poppy
Seed Dressing & Hazelnuts

Raw Satay Salad

Grilled Courgette &
Asparagus Salad with
Orange Dressing

NUTTY WILD RICE SALAD

This flavoursome, nutty salad is full of fibre and protein.
It's super-fresh tasting and one of my favourites!

SERVES 4 GENEROUSLY

250g (2 cups) wild rice

30g (1/4 cup) coconut flakes

30g (1/4 cup) hazelnuts

30g (1/4 cup) pecans

4 spring onions (scallions),
finely chopped

45g (1/4 cup) dried
apricots, chopped

1/2 green (bell) pepper, cubed

140g (3/4 cup) canned
sweetcorn, drained

a few fresh mint leaves, chopped

juice of 1 lime

2 tbsp hazelnut oil

pinch salt

pinch cayenne pepper

pinch dried chilli flakes

Cook the rice according to the packet instructions. Once cooked, run cold water over the rice to cool it completely.

While the rice is cooking, toast the coconut flakes and nuts in a dry frying pan on the hob or on a baking tray in an oven heated to 180°C (350°F) for 5 minutes, until lightly toasted. Keep a close eye on them so they don't burn! Set aside to cool.

Once the rice and nuts are cool, add them to a large bowl with the rest of the ingredients. Mix thoroughly and serve chilled.

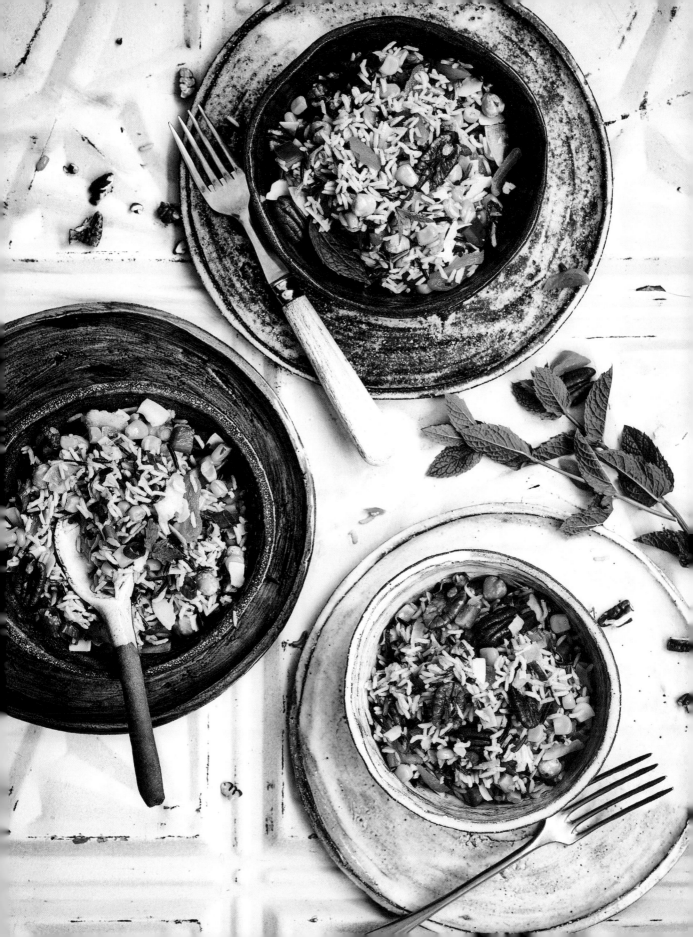

ASPARAGUS
& KALE CAESAR SALAD

I've veganized this classic salad and added a slight twist: grilled ciabatta and a sprinkle of coconut "bacon" bits. It's creamy and delicious.

SERVES 4

10 asparagus tips

handful of kale, shredded

130g (1 cup) frozen peas

1 tbsp olive oil

4 slices of ciabatta

2 heads of baby gem, leaves separated and washed

a few fresh mint leaves

a few fresh dill leaves

coconut "bacon" (see page 124)

For the dressing:

1 garlic clove, crushed

1 tbsp capers, finely chopped

4 tbsp "Mayonnaise" (see page 24)

2 tbsp nutritional yeast

1 tbsp fresh lemon juice

pinch sea salt and pepper

Preheat the oven to 180°C (350°F) and line a baking tray with greaseproof paper. Fill a bowl full of iced water.

Meanwhile, bring a large saucepan of water to a rolling boil, add a pinch of sea salt, then add the asparagus, shortly followed by the kale and peas. Cook for no more than 60 seconds then remove from the water and submerge into the bowl of ice-cold water, so they stop cooking immediately. When cold, remove from the water, drain and set aside.

Heat a griddle pan over a high heat, add a tablespoon of olive oil and, when the pan is hot, grill the sliced ciabatta. Try and get some nice charred lines on each side, then remove from the pan. Cut into smaller pieces.

Mix all of the dressing ingredients together in a small bowl until well incorporated.

Toss the lettuce, asparagus, kale, peas and herbs in a small amount of the dressing in a serving bowl. Scatter the coconut bacon and grilled ciabatta on top, and the rest of the dressing alongside.

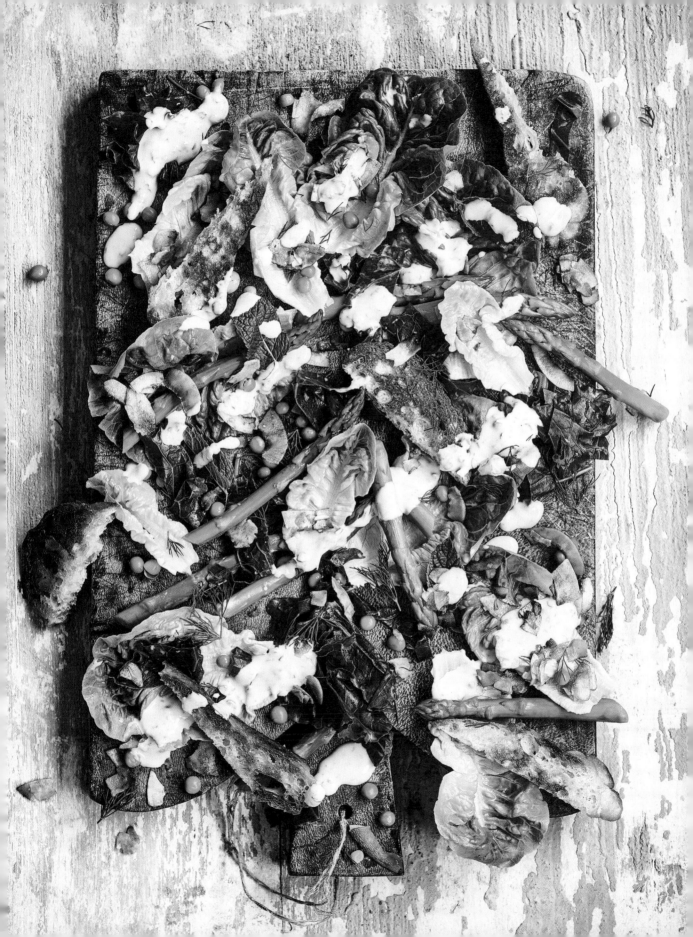

BEETROOT, SWEET POTATO, ORANGE & WALNUT SALAD

This warm salad tastes as good as it looks; it's so vibrant! The earthy, sweet beetroot works very well with the tangy dressing and the walnuts add a beautiful crunch. It's the perfect autumn salad.

SERVES 4

3 beetroots (beets), peeled

2 sweet potatoes, peeled

1 tbsp olive oil

2 sprigs fresh thyme

2 oranges, peeled and sliced

handful of rocket (arugula)

handful of spinach

3 tbsp chopped chives

30g (¼ cup) walnuts, lightly toasted in a dry pan

For the dressing:

3 tbsp walnut oil or extra virgin olive oil

1 tsp wholegrain mustard

2 tbsp red wine vinegar

zest of ½ orange

pinch salt and pepper

Preheat the oven to 200°C (400°F). Line a baking tray with greaseproof paper.

Cut the beetroot and sweet potato into evenly sized wedges. Transfer them to the baking tray, drizzle with the olive oil and give it a good mix to make sure all the pieces are coated. Break up the fresh thyme in your hands and add to the tray. Bake for 25 minutes, or until soft.

Mix the dressing ingredients together in a small bowl.

Once the potato and beetroot are cooked, remove from the oven and allow to cool slightly.

Add the orange slices, rocket, spinach, chives and walnuts to a serving bowl, followed by the warm beetroot and potato. Drizzle over a couple tablespoons of the dressing, mix lightly and serve straight away.

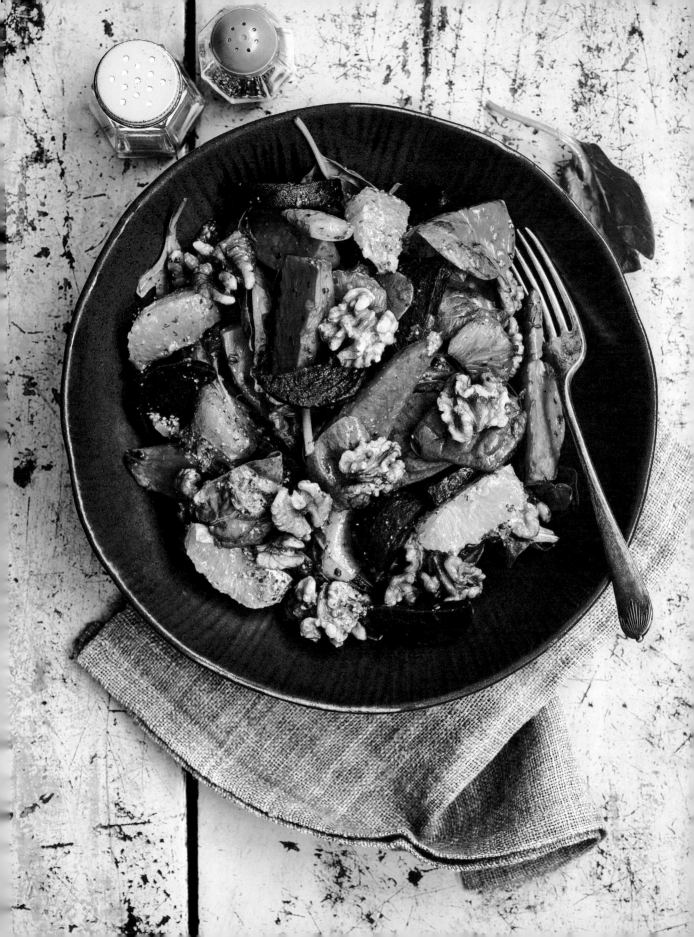

RAW ROOT SALAD WITH POPPY SEED DRESSING & HAZELNUTS

This raw salad has intense flavours and the dressing enhances the amazing natural sweetness of the raw vegetables. Use different varieties of beetroot – golden, red and "chioggia" – to make it even more colourful.

SERVES 4

3 mixed beetroots (beets)

1 small celeriac (celery root)

2 carrots

1 sweet apple

4 radishes

2 spring onions (scallions)

4 tbsp pomegranate seeds

3 tbsp raw hazelnuts, chopped

2 tbsp fresh tarragon, chopped

For the dressing:

1 tbsp poppy seeds

4 tbsp apple cider vinegar

2 tbsp agave nectar

2 tbsp fresh orange juice

pinch sea salt and pepper

Peel the beetroots, then use a mandoline set on its thinnest setting to slice them into discs into a large mixing bowl. If you don't have a mandoline, peel the flesh with a vegetable peeler to get long ribbons.

Peel the celeriac, then continue to peel the flesh to get really nice long ribbons. Do the same with the carrots, then add both to the bowl.

Slice the apple, radishes and spring onions as thinly as possible with a sharp knife and add to the bowl with the pomegranate seeds.

To make the dressing, simply combine all the ingredients together in a small bowl.

Pour all of the dressing over the vegetables, mix well then chill in the fridge for at least 15 minutes. The acidity in the dressing softens the vegetables and intensifies the flavours.

Serve with a sprinkling of chopped hazelnuts and tarragon.

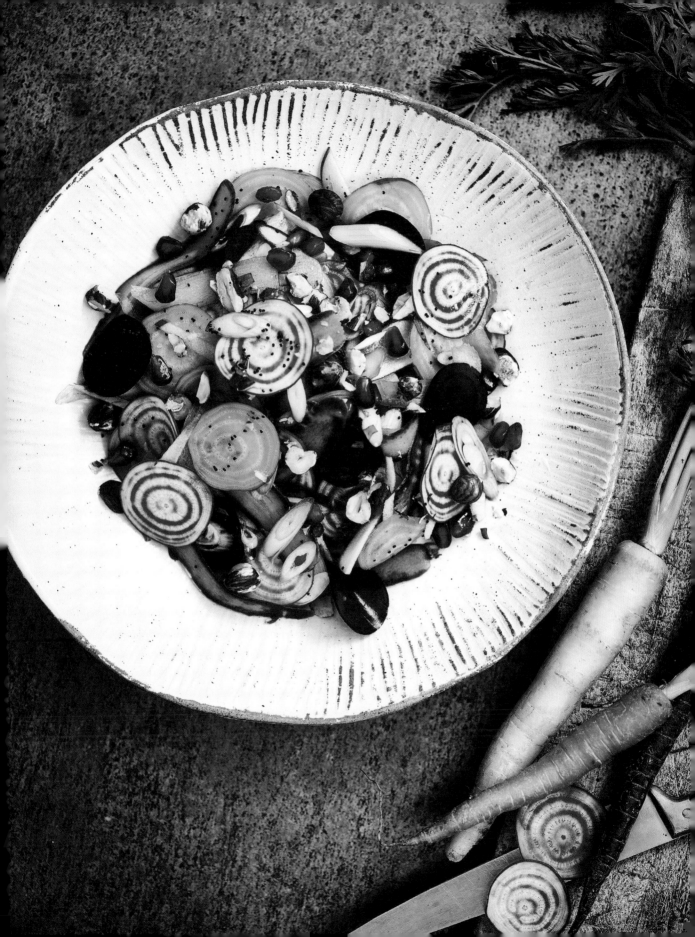

RAW SATAY SALAD

This raw salad has the perfect blend of flavours: sweet, spicy, fresh and nutty. I love these Asian notes. The edamame and peanuts are great sources of protein.

SERVES 6

3 carrots, grated

1 courgette (zucchini), grated

75g (1 cup) finely shredded red cabbage

110g (1 cup) frozen edamame, defrosted

handful of pea shoots

15g (2 sprigs) Thai basil, leaves picked

55g ($\frac{1}{2}$ cup) sugar snap peas, split in half

2 heads of gem lettuce

For the dressing:

2 tbsp Peanut & Almond Butter (see page 33)

1 garlic clove, crushed

1 small red chilli, deseeded and finely chopped

3-cm ($1\frac{1}{2}$-inch) piece of fresh ginger, finely chopped

2 tbsp light soy sauce

1 tbsp maple syrup or coconut sugar

2 tbsp fresh lime juice

2 tsp tahini

120ml ($\frac{1}{2}$ cup) water

2 tbsp mixed sesame seeds

First make the dressing: whisk together all of the ingredients in a bowl or jug and set aside.

Add the salad ingredients to a serving bowl, toss together then pour over the dressing and mix well. Serve straight away.

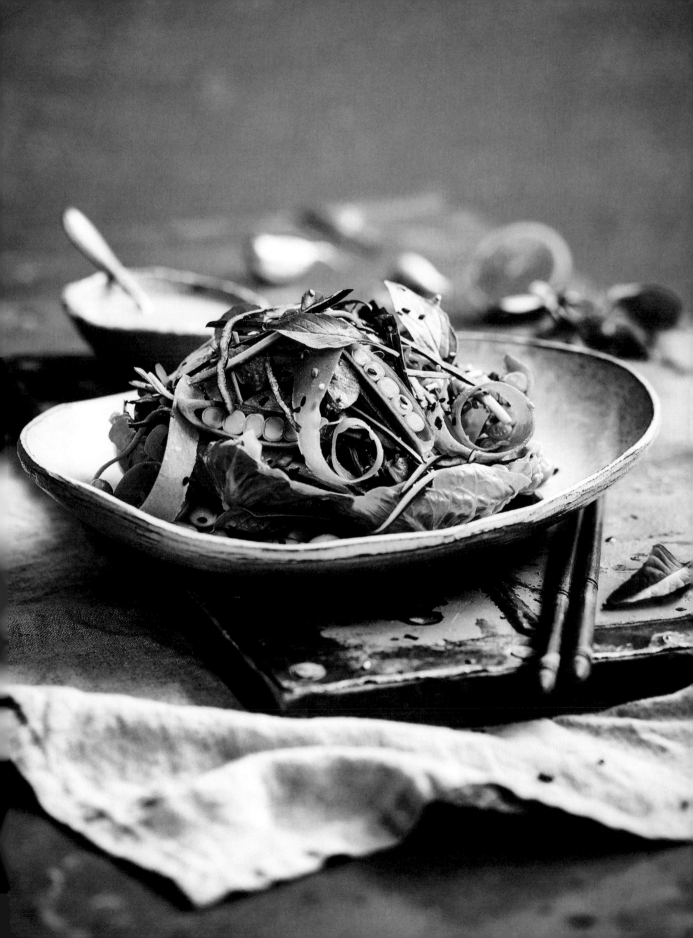

GRILLED COURGETTE & ASPARAGUS SALAD WITH ORANGE DRESSING

This salad came about through my love for spring/summer ingredients: asparagus, samphire, courgettes, watercress... The list goes on. The charring on the courgette gives the salad a new dimension of flavour which is simply amazing!

SERVES 4

250g (2 cups) asparagus tips

35g (¹/₂ cup) samphire

35g (¹/₂ cup) broad beans, peeled

35g (¹/₂ cup) peas

1 tsp olive oil

1 courgette (zucchini), sliced very thinly lengthways

60g (3 cups) fresh watercress

35g (¹/₂ cup) sugar snap peas

handful of fresh mint leaves

2 tbsp toasted pistachios

2 tbsp toasted pine nuts

For the dressing:

juice and zest ¹/₂ orange

juice ¹/₂ lime

1 tsp dried chilli flakes

2 tbsp extra virgin olive oil

pinch sea salt

pinch cracked black pepper

First up, fill a large bowl with cold water and add a handful of ice cubes.

Bring a large saucepan of water to a rolling boil. Add a pinch of salt, then the asparagus tips. Cook for 30 seconds before adding the samphire, broad beans and peas. After 30 seconds remove everything from the boiling water and quickly plunge it all into the bowl of ice-cold water. After a minute in the cold water, remove all the vegetables and set aside on a plate lined with kitchen paper to drain. You should have super-green, tender asparagus with a beautiful bite to it, so make sure you don't over-cook it.

Preheat a griddle pan, add the olive oil, then grill the courgette slices on each side until charred.

Meanwhile, mix together all the dressing ingredients in a bowl.

Now it's time to construct the salad! Grab a big mixing bowl, add the watercress, sugar snaps and mint leaves, then the blanched asparagus, samphire, broad beans and peas, the toasted nuts and chargrilled courgette. Drizzle over the beautiful dressing and give it a good mix to combine.

Serve up on a big plate and dig in!

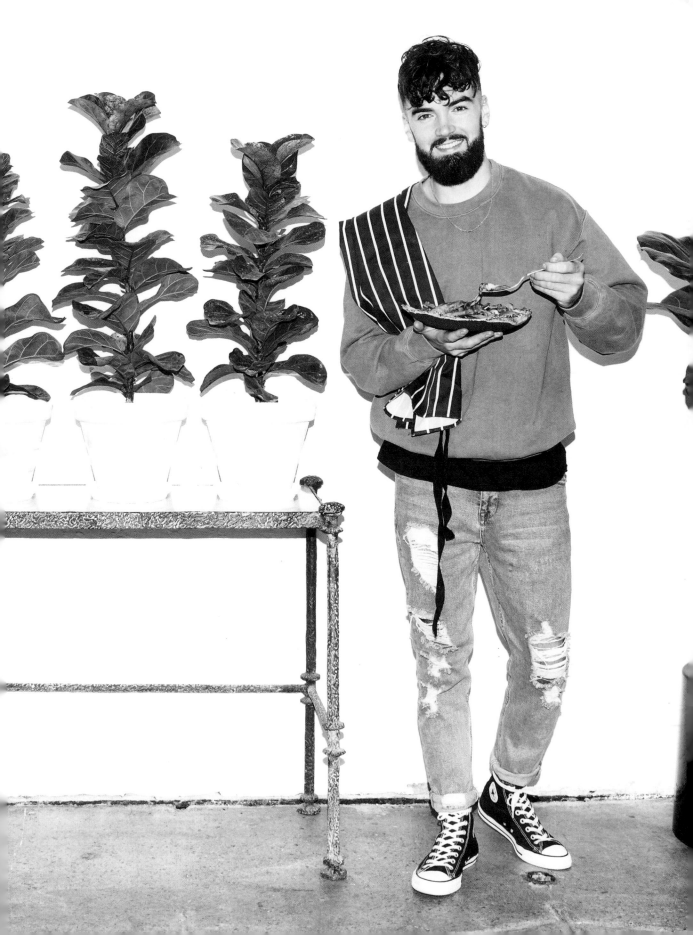

SIDES

Classic Tempura Vegetables
with Dipping Sauce

Sweet Potato Fries

Rainbow Slaw

Mixed Lemon Greens

Gravy Goals

"Bake-In-A-Bag"
Moroccan-Style Vegetables

Dauphinoise Potatoes

Herb & Lemon Polenta Chips

CLASSIC TEMPURA VEGETABLES
WITH DIPPING SAUCE

Definitely an occasional treat. You may think covering your vegetables in a batter then deep-frying would spoil them but this classic tempura recipe celebrates the vegetables beautifully. Make sure the batter is really light and your oil is hot, so they cook quickly and don't lose flavour.

SERVES 4

handful of asparagus tips

1 carrot, peeled and sliced into 4-mm ($\frac{1}{8}$-inch) discs

1 red onion, quartered

handful of kale leaves

1 head of broccoli, separated into florets

1 litre (4 cups) vegetable oil, for frying

For the batter:

65g ($\frac{1}{2}$ cup) plain (all-purpose) flour (or gluten-free flour)

65g ($\frac{1}{2}$ cup) cornflour (cornstarch)

pinch sea salt

240ml (1 cup) sparkling water

For the dipping sauce:

2 tbsp rice wine vinegar

2 tbsp light soy sauce

1 tsp dried chilli flakes

1 tsp maple syrup

1 small garlic clove, crushed

Preheat a deep-fat fryer filled with the oil to 180°C (350°F), or half-fill a large saucepan with oil and put on a medium heat.

Mix all the dipping sauce ingredients together in a small bowl and set aside.

Add the flours and salt to a large mixing bowl and combine. Whisk in the water gradually until you have a very light, loose batter. (The batter will only just coat the vegetables.)

Dip the vegetables into the batter, one at a time, shake off any excess, then transfer carefully to the hot oil. Don't over-crowd the fryer or saucepan – it's best to fry just a few pieces at a time.

Fry the vegetables for 2–3 minutes, then remove using a spider strainer or slotted spoon and place onto a kitchen paper-lined baking tray to drain the excess oil. Transfer to a low oven with the door open to keep warm while you fry the rest.

Serve straight away with the dipping sauce.

SWEET POTATO FRIES

Follow this recipe to make crispy sweet potato fries in the oven. Sweet potato fries are the healthy option when you're craving chips, and the fact that these are oven-baked makes them even healthier.

SERVES 4

2 sweet potatoes, peeled and cut into 5-mm ($\frac{1}{4}$-inch) chips

$\frac{1}{2}$ tsp paprika

$\frac{1}{2}$ tsp cayenne pepper

$\frac{1}{2}$ tsp dried oregano

1 tsp sea salt

$\frac{1}{2}$ tsp cracked black pepper

4 garlic cloves, bruised (optional)

2 sprigs thyme (optional)

3 tbsp extra virgin olive oil

Preheat the oven to 180°C (350°F). Line a large baking tray with greaseproof paper.

Put the potatoes, spices, seasoning – including the garlic and thyme, if using – and oil into a large mixing bowl and toss really well to make sure all the chips are well coated.

Spread the coated chips out on the lined baking tray, making sure they are in a single layer and not stacked on top of each other.

Bake in the oven for 30 minutes, turning over halfway through cooking to make sure the fries cook evenly.

Serve them straight away. (They go very well with my BBQ Sauce on page 24.)

RAINBOW SLAW

This colourful slaw is an amazing addition to many meals, especially the Jackfruit Lettuce Wraps (see page 105) and Quarter Pounders (see page 111).

SERVES 3–4

100g (2 cups) finely shredded red cabbage

3 carrots, peeled and grated

1 red onion, finely sliced

handful of coriander (cilantro), finely chopped

6 tbsp "Mayonnaise" (see page 24)

pinch sea salt and pepper

Combine all the ingredients in a large mixing bowl and mix well. Check for seasoning, then serve.

MIXED LEMON GREENS

An excellent nutritious addition to any meal. Be sure to only briefly boil the vegetables – it would be a huge shame to over-cook them. Try this same recipe with asparagus or mangetout.

SERVES 3–4

200g (7oz) Tenderstem broccoli, ends trimmed

200g (7oz) cavolo nero, stems removed and shredded

100g (3$\frac{1}{2}$oz) spring greens, shredded

zest and juice of $\frac{1}{2}$ lemon

pinch sea salt and pepper

Bring a large saucepan three-quarters full of water to a fast boil. Add a pinch of sea salt, then drop in the broccoli and cook for about 60 seconds with the lid on. Then add the cavolo nero and spring greens, and cook with the lid on for 30 seconds more.

Quickly remove the vegetables from the water, drain and transfer to a mixing bowl. Add the lemon juice and zest and season with salt and pepper. Toss everything together and serve straight away.

GRAVY GOALS

Packed full of assertive flavour, this gravy is as bold as any I've come across. It goes really well with the Wellington (see page 138) and the Ultimate Vegan Roast (see page 141).

SERVES 4-5

2 carrots, peeled

2 red onions, peeled

250g (2 cups) chestnut mushrooms

2 garlic cloves

1 leek, washed

2 sticks of celery, washed

1 tbsp olive oil

pinch sea salt and pepper

2 tbsp plain (all-purpose) flour (or gluten-free flour)

120ml ($\frac{1}{2}$ cup) red wine

1 tbsp soy sauce

1 tbsp Marmite

1 tbsp balsamic vinegar

2 sprigs fresh thyme

2 sprigs fresh sage

1 sprig fresh rosemary

720ml (3 cups) Vegetable Stock (see page 31)

Roughly chop the carrots, onions, mushrooms, garlic, leek and celery.

Heat a large saucepan over a medium heat and add the olive oil. When the pan is hot, add the onions and mushrooms. Sauté for 2 minutes until they've shrunk in size. Add the rest of the vegetables and a pinch of seasoning, and continue to sauté for 3 minutes, stirring often.

Let the veg go golden and caramelize nicely but make sure they don't burn. Stir in the flour and cook for 1 minute more.

Pour in the red wine to deglaze the pan, then reduce the heat to low. Next add the soy sauce, Marmite and balsamic vinegar.

Give everything a good stir, then add the herbs. Allow the flavours to intensify for 2 minutes before adding the vegetable stock.

It's now time to leave the gravy to simmer and reduce down for 15 minutes.

After 15 minutes the gravy should be a lot thicker. Pass the gravy through a fine sieve into a small saucepan, pressing as much of the liquid out of the vegetables as you can using the back of a ladle.

Serve the gravy straight away, or if it's still slightly thin let it reduce for a few more minutes.

Cool and freeze any excess gravy for use another day.

"BAKE-IN-A-BAG" MOROCCAN-STYLE VEGETABLES

I love this method of cooking as the flavours can't escape; the vegetables almost steam-roast inside the bag and create a beautiful sauce. Ras el hanout – a mixture of several ground spices – is a favourite spice mix of mine. The name's translation from Arabic is "head of the shop", an expression which actually means "the best of the shop".

SERVES 4

1 small butternut squash
(leave the peel on)

2 red onions

1 red (bell) pepper

2 courgettes (zucchinis)

1 aubergine (eggplant)

200g (2 cups) cherry tomatoes

8 garlic cloves

4 sprigs fresh thyme

2 sprigs fresh rosemary

2 tbsp ras el hanout

pinch sea salt and pepper

3 tbsp extra virgin
olive oil (optional)

Preheat the oven to 180°C (350°F). Prepare 4 large sheets of foil and greaseproof paper.

Slice the squash in 2, deseed and cut the flesh into even-sized chunks of around 2cm (³/₄ inch). Place the squash in a large mixing bowl.

Peel and slice the onions into 8 pieces. Cube the peppers, courgettes and aubergine into even-sized chunks, then add them all to the bowl.

Remove any stalks from the cherry tomatoes. Add these to the bowl with the garlic (which you don't even have to peel), thyme and rosemary.

Sprinkle over the ras el hanout and seasoning, and mix everything together with your hands.

Divide into 4 and make sure you have a good mixture of each type of veg. Spoon into the middle of a piece of greaseproof paper and drizzle over some oil (if using). Gather the corners of the paper together and twist to secure the vegetables inside. Lift the package onto the foil sheet and wrap up tightly. Repeat the process for the rest of the vegetables until you have 4 parcels.

Place onto a baking tray, then bake in the oven for 35 minutes.

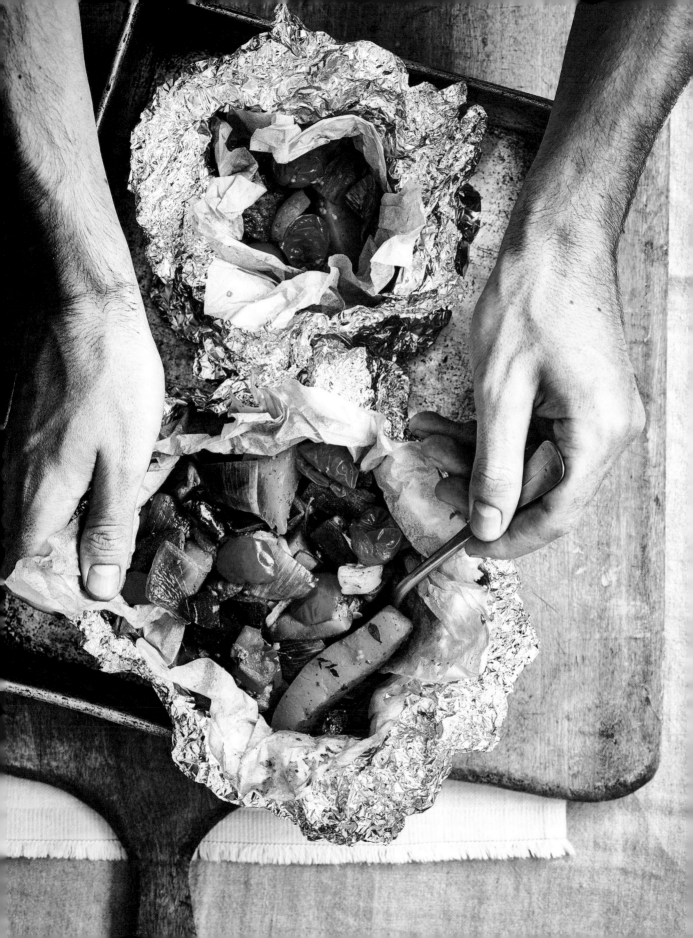

DAUPHINOISE POTATOES

This dish was one of my favourite treats before becoming vegan but this version actually tastes better than the original. That's the magic of coconut milk! It's also a lot less time-consuming and the mustard adds a little umami.

SERVES 5

6 Maris Piper potatoes, peeled

5 shallots

1 x 400-ml (14-oz) can coconut milk

250ml (1 cup) soy milk

4 garlic cloves, crushed

3 sprigs fresh thyme

1 bay leaf

3 tbsp wholegrain mustard

2 tbsp nutritional yeast

pinch sea salt and pepper

Preheat the oven to 190°C (375°F).

Slice the potatoes very finely using a mandoline or food processor, on the finest setting. Finely slice the shallots with a sharp knife.

Pour the coconut and soy milk into a large saucepan and add the garlic, thyme, bay leaf, mustard, yeast and seasoning.

Heat until boiling, then add the sliced potatoes and onions and stir gently. Remove from the heat and pour carefully into a shallow 1.5-litre (2$\frac{1}{2}$-pint) ovenproof dish (I sometimes use a 20-cm [8-inch] square oven dish). Spread the potato out so it's compact and level, then cover with a sheet of greaseproof paper.

Bake for 20 minutes before removing the paper and baking for a further 20 minutes.

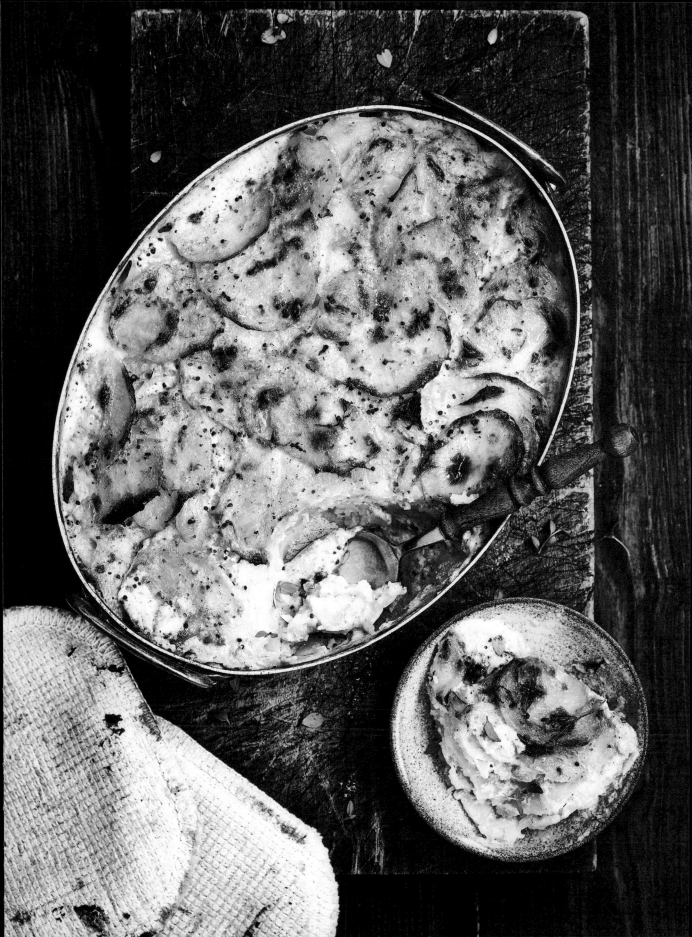

HERB & LEMON POLENTA CHIPS

Polenta is an amazing source of calcium, magnesium and fibre – and these "chips" jazz up the rather bland flavour. They're great alongside the Quarter Pounders (see page 111).

SERVES 3–4

400ml (2 cups) Vegetable Stock (see page 31)

150g (1 cup) fine instant polenta

pinch sea salt and pepper

2 tbsp herbes de provence

zest of 1 lemon

2 tbsp extra virgin olive oil

Line a 3-cm (1-inch) deep, 20-cm (8-inch) square baking tray with greaseproof paper, leaving excess paper hanging over the sides.

Pour the vegetable stock into a medium saucepan and bring to a boil. Whisk in the polenta and keep whisking for around 2 minutes, until the mixture starts to thicken. Once thickened, remove the pan from the heat, add the seasoning, herbs and lemon zest and stir well.

Pour the mixture into the lined baking tray and smooth flat with a spatula, then chill in the fridge to set for around 2 hours.

Preheat the oven to 180°C (350°F) and remove the polenta from the fridge. Lift the firm block of polenta out of the tray using the overhanging paper as handles. Cut the polenta into chunky chips, brush with the olive oil, scatter on a baking tray, then bake in the oven for 20–25 minutes, or until golden. Season with salt and pepper then serve straight away.

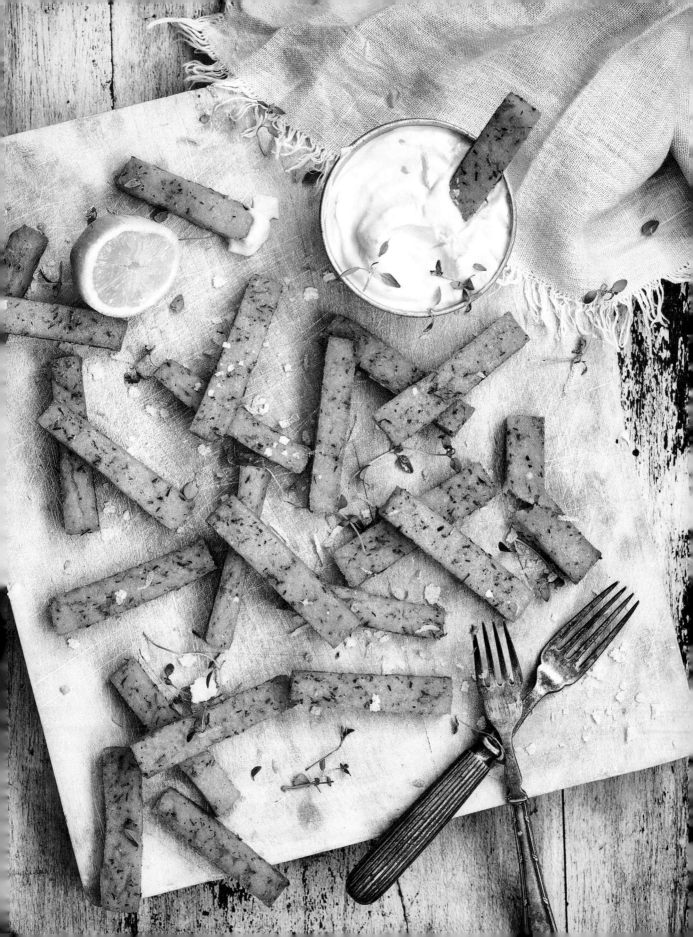

BREAD OF HEAVEN

Pretzel-Style Burger Buns

Beer Hot Dog Rolls

Vine Tomato, Basil &
Rosemary Focaccia

Grilled Flatbreads

Basic Pizza Dough & Sauce

You-Won't-Believe-It's-
Gluten-Free Loaf

PRETZEL-STYLE BURGER BUNS

**Light and soft inside with that nice chewy outer crust,
these pretzel-style burger buns are perfect with any burger.**

MAKES 6 LARGE BUNS

8g (¼oz) active dried yeast

240ml (1 cup) lukewarm
water, plus a little extra

500g (3½ cups) strong
white bread flour

pinch sea salt

50g (¼ cup) vegan
"butter", melted

2 tbsp dark brown soft sugar

For the glaze:

1 tbsp almond milk

1 tbsp extra virgin olive oil

2 tsp agave nectar

1 tsp rock salt

Line 2 baking trays with
greaseproof paper.

First up, make the dough – it
couldn't be simpler! Mix the yeast
and lukewarm water together in
a mixing jug. Leave for around
10 minutes, until slightly bubbly.

Meanwhile, weigh out the flour
and salt in a large mixing bowl. Add
the melted butter to the water and
yeast mixture. Make a well in the
flour and add the yeast and butter
mixture and the sugar.

Stir until the dough starts coming
together – get your hands involved.
(You'll get them messy, but it's
worth it!)

Once all the ingredients have come together, tip the dough onto a lightly floured work surface. Now it's time to knead, so roll up your sleeves and work that dough. You want to knead for around 10 minutes, after which the dough should be smooth and quite elastic.

Lightly oil your mixing bowl and lift the dough back into it. The oil will prevent the dough from sticking. Lay a clean, damp tea towel over the top of the bowl and leave somewhere warm for around 1 hour, or until the dough has doubled in size.

After 1 hour, remove the dough from the bowl; it should feel beautiful and light. (I love this part...) Knock back the dough (which basically means to knock the air out of it) and knead it for around 4 more minutes.

Divide the dough into around 6 evenly sized pieces and roll each piece into a ball. Arrange the rolls on the lined baking trays, making sure you leave at least 3cm (1 inch) between each roll.

Cover the trays with damp tea towels and place the trays somewhere warm for an hour, or until doubled in size.

Preheat the oven to 200°C (400°F) and place an empty roasting tray on the bottom shelf or base of the oven.

Mix the glaze ingredients (excluding the salt) together in a small bowl.

Remove the tea towel from the rolls, brush them with the glaze and sprinkle a little rock salt on top of each one. You can score a couple of lines on the top, too, if you wish.

Pour a cup of water into the empty baking tray inside the oven to create steam when the buns are cooking (which will give you light, soft buns).

Bake the buns for 20 minutes, or until golden. Remove from the oven when cooked and transfer to a wire rack to cool.

Store the buns in a sealed plastic sandwich bag.

BEER HOT DOG ROLLS

The added yeasty flavour and bubbles in the beer make the taste of these hot dog rolls the best ever. They go so well with the Chilli Dogs on page 108.

MAKES 6 LARGE ROLLS

120ml ($^{1}/_{2}$ cup) almond Milk (see page 12)

120ml ($^{1}/_{2}$ cup) vegan-friendly ale

8g ($^{1}/_{4}$oz) active dried yeast

50g ($^{1}/_{4}$ cup) vegan "butter", melted

500g ($3^{1}/_{2}$ cups) strong white bread flour

pinch sea salt

2 tbsp dark brown soft sugar

For the glaze:

2 tbsp almond Milk (see page 12)

2 tbsp extra virgin olive oil

1 tbsp agave nectar

1 tsp rock salt

1 tsp poppy seeds

Line 2 baking trays with greaseproof paper.

Mix the milk and ale together in a small saucepan and heat until the mixture is lukewarm. Remove the pan from the heat and whisk in the yeast. Leave for around 10 minutes, until slightly bubbly, then add the melted butter.

Meanwhile, place the flour and salt in a large mixing bowl. When the milk/yeast mixture is ready, make a well in the middle of the flour and pour it in with the sugar, stirring to combine.

Once the dough comes together, tip it out onto a lightly floured work surface. Now it's time to knead.

You want to knead for around 10 minutes, after which the dough should be smooth and quite elastic, and smell super-yeasty! Lightly oil your mixing bowl and lift the dough back into it. The oil will prevent the dough from sticking. Lay a clean, damp tea towel over the top of the bowl and leave somewhere warm for around 1 hour, or until the dough has doubled in size.

After an hour, remove the dough from the bowl (it should feel beautiful and light), knock it back and knead for around 4 more minutes.

Divide the dough into around 6 pieces and roll each into a sausage/mini baguette shape. Arrange the rolls on the lined baking trays, making sure you leave at least 3cm (1 inch) between each roll. Cover the trays with damp tea towels and place somewhere warm for 1 hour, or until doubled in size.

Preheat the oven to 200°C (400°F) and place an empty roasting tray on the bottom shelf.

Mix the glaze ingredients, apart from the salt and poppy seeds, together in a small bowl.

Remove the tea towel from the rolls, score a couple of lines on the top of each roll with a sharp knife, then brush the tops with the glaze and sprinkle over the rock salt and poppy seeds.

Pour a cup of water into the empty tray inside the oven to create steam when the rolls are cooking (to give you light, soft rolls) and bake the rolls for 20–25 minutes, or until golden. Remove from the oven when cooked and transfer to a wire rack to cool.

Store the rolls in a sealed plastic sandwich bag.

VINE TOMATO, BASIL & ROSEMARY FOCACCIA

Focaccia is one of the simplest breads to make and, in my opinion, one of the tastiest. I have simplified a traditional recipe, so a cook of any skill level will be able to make this. I've also added wholemeal flour. Make sure you press the tomatoes and herbs into the dough so the flavour runs right through.

SERVES ABOUT 5

2 tsp active dried yeast

2 tbsp extra virgin olive oil

280ml (2 cups) lukewarm water

290g (2½ cups) strong white bread flour

290g (2½ cups) wholemeal flour

pinch sea salt

Topping suggestions:

3 bunches of vine cherry tomatoes

handful of fresh basil leaves

2 sprigs fresh rosemary

½ tsp sea salt flakes

1 tsp smoked chilli flakes (optional)

2–3 tbsp olive oil, smoked if you can find it

Line a large baking dish or tray with baking paper.

Mix the yeast and olive oil into the lukewarm water and leave for around 10 minutes, until slightly bubbly.

Meanwhile, place the flours and salt in a large mixing bowl. Make a well in the centre of the flours, then add the water and yeast mix and stir until the dough starts to come together.

Tip the dough onto a lightly floured work surface and knead for around 10 minutes. The dough should then be smooth and quite elastic.

Lightly oil your mixing bowl and lift the dough back into it. The oil will prevent the dough from sticking. Lay a clean, damp tea towel over the top of the bowl and leave somewhere warm for around 1 hour, or until the dough has doubled in size.

After an hour, remove the dough from the bowl, knock it back and knead for around 5 more minutes.

Then place the dough in the lined baking dish or tray and pull/shape the dough into the shape of your choice – I like a rustic look. Make sure it's around 1.5cm (½ inch) thick. Place a damp tea towel over the top and leave to rise again, this time for 30 minutes.

Preheat the oven to 200°C (400°F).

When the focaccia has proved for a second time, press the tomatoes, basil and rosemary into the dough. Be firm – press the toppings deep into the dough, so that when it cooks the flavours are running right through the bread. Sprinkle over the salt and chilli flakes (if using), and a good drizzle of olive oil. Bake for 35 minutes, then serve straight away.

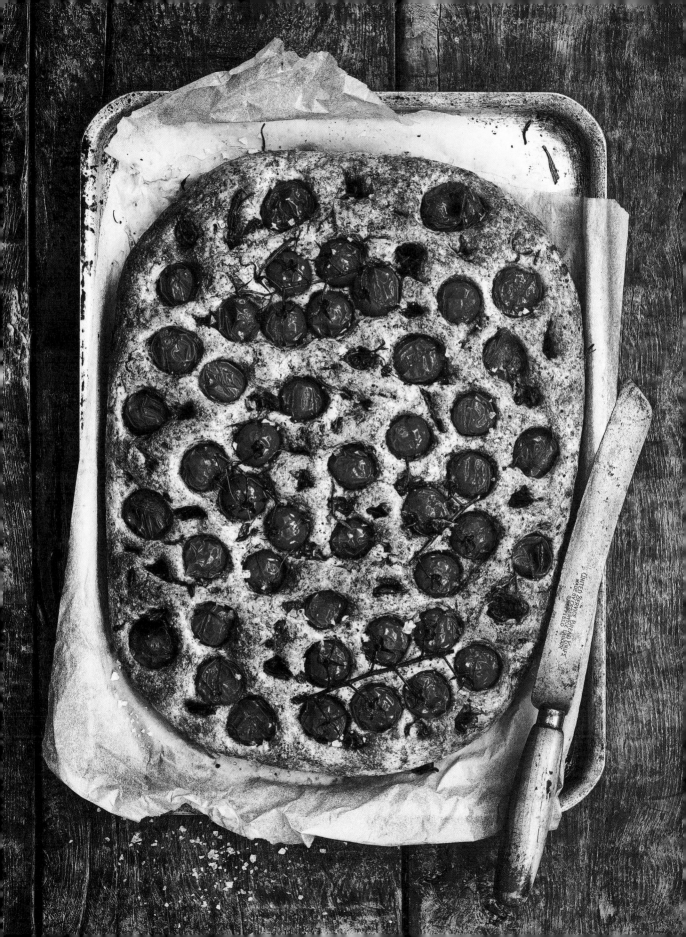

GRILLED FLATBREADS

These flatbreads are a delight and take just 30 minutes to make!
Make sure your griddle pan is smoking hot – you want to get some charring
on those flatbreads. Serve as wraps; or they're perfect with
falafel (see page 88), tagines and so much more.

MAKES 8

300g (2½ cups) self-raising flour

2 pinches sea salt

1 tsp baking powder

1 tsp paprika

300g (1¼ cups) coconut yogurt

2 tbsp chilli olive oil

handful of fresh parsley,
chopped (optional)

Mix the flour, a pinch of salt, the baking powder and paprika together in a large mixing bowl. Pour in the coconut yogurt and mix together with a spatula.

Once the dough has come together in a ball, turn it out onto a lightly floured work surface and knead for around 8 minutes.

Return the dough to the bowl, cover with a damp tea towel and leave to rest for 10 minutes.

Once rested, cut the dough into 8 pieces. Using your hands or a rolling pin, roll the dough out into a rough circle approximately 1cm (½ inch) thick.

Preheat a griddle pan over a high heat. Turn the extractor fan on and open the windows – the key is to get the pan super-hot! Add a small amount of the chilli oil and grill each flatbread individually for 2 minutes on each side. They should fluff up beautifully while cooking. Repeat until you've grilled all the flatbreads, adding a little more oil to the pan, then sprinkle over some fresh parsley and a pinch of salt before serving.

BASIC PIZZA DOUGH & SAUCE

Whether you cook your pizza in a wood-fired oven or a conventional oven, this pizza dough will produce the perfect pizza every time. The tangy tomato sauce is a winner, too.

MAKES ENOUGH FOR 6 PIZZAS

For the pizza dough:

300ml (1¼ cups) lukewarm water

2 tsp active dried yeast

500g (3½ cups) 00 flour (or strong white bread flour), plus extra for dusting

pinch sea salt

3 tbsp extra virgin olive oil

For the tomato sauce:

1 tbsp extra virgin olive oil

1 onion, chopped

1 garlic clove, crushed

1 x 400-g (14-oz) can chopped tomatoes

1 tbsp tomato puree

handful of fresh oregano

pinch sea salt and pepper

To make the pizza dough, mix together the lukewarm water and yeast in a jug and set aside for 5 minutes to activate the yeast.

In a large mixing bowl, mix together the flour and salt. Make a well in the middle, add the olive oil to the yeast mixture, then pour into the flour. Stir with your hands until it starts to come together; the mix will feel quite wet at first.

Sprinkle flour onto a clean work surface and turn the dough out onto it. Knead the dough for around 10 minutes, adding additional flour if you need to.

Once kneaded the dough will feel lovely and smooth. Portion the dough into 6, then form into balls. Place the dough balls onto a lightly oiled baking tray, then cover the tray with a damp tea towel and leave to rise for at least 1 hour, or until doubled in size.

Meanwhile, make the tomato sauce: heat the olive oil in a saucepan, then sauté the onion and garlic until golden. Add the tomatoes and tomato puree and stir well. Simmer for 5 minutes before adding the oregano and some seasoning.

Roughly blitz the sauce with a hand-held blender. Use the sauce to top your pizzas, store in the fridge until needed, or freeze.

Preheat the oven to 200°C (400°F).

Once the dough has risen, roll it out into pizzas approximately 3mm (⅛ inch) thick, transfer to a baking sheet, spoon tomato sauce on top, and add any extra toppings of your choice.

Bake for 12 minutes, until turning golden at the edges.

YOU-WON'T-BELIEVE-IT'S-GLUTEN-FREE LOAF

This bread is almost unrecognizable as gluten free – it has a beautiful nutty flavour and the texture is surprisingly light.

MAKES 1 LOAF

180ml (³/₄ cup) lukewarm water

120ml (¹/₂ cup) lukewarm almond Milk (see page 12)

2 tsp active dried yeast

3 tbsp extra virgin olive oil

90g (³/₄ cup) buckwheat flour

135g (1 cup) rice flour

135g (1 cup) oat flour (or blended rolled oats)

55g (¹/₂ cup) tapioca starch

1 tsp baking powder

¹/₂ tsp bicarbonate of soda (baking soda)

1 tbsp raw brown sugar

1 tsp sea salt

2 tbsp Egg Replacement (see page 32)

Line a 450-g (1-lb) loaf tin with greaseproof paper.

Mix the lukewarm water and milk with the yeast and olive oil in a mixing jug. Leave for around 5 minutes, until slightly bubbly.

Meanwhile, sift all the flours together with the starch, baking powder, bicarbonate of soda, sugar and salt into a large mixing bowl and mix together thoroughly. I sift the mix together at least 3 times.

Make a well in the middle of the flour mixture and pour in the water and yeast mixture, and the egg replacement. Stir until the dough starts to come together.

Once you have a ball of dough, tip it out onto a lightly floured work surface. Now it's time to knead: knead for around 5 minutes. If your dough feels too wet, add a touch

more rice flour to the surface. Place the dough into the lined loaf tin, and press the dough into the corners of the tin.

Lay a clean, damp tea towel over the top of the dough and leave it somewhere warm for around 1 hour, or until the dough has doubled in size.

Preheat the oven to 180°C (350°F).

Once the dough has doubled in size and your oven is hot, place the tin into the oven on the middle shelf to bake for 1 hour. When cooked the loaf should have a nice golden crust and sound hollow when you tap it.

Allow to cool a little, then remove from the tin and transfer to a wire rack to cool completely before slicing.

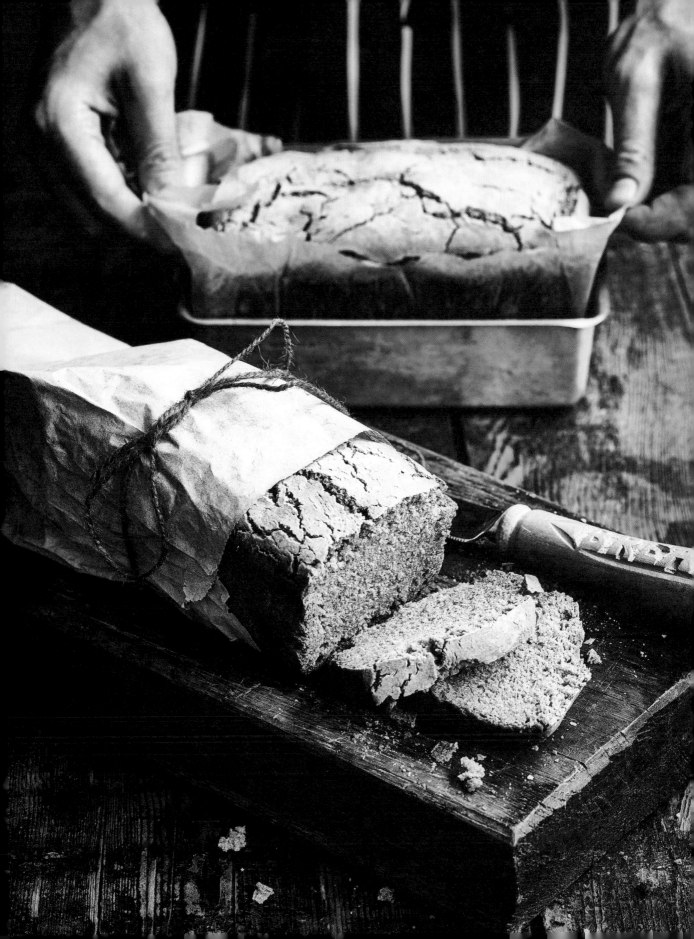

SWEET TALKING

Mint, Choc Chip
& Matcha Ice Cream

Raw Mango & Vanilla
Ice Cream

Lemon "Meringue" Pie

Chocolate Fondants

Fancy Baked Doughnuts

Salted-Caramel Pretzel,
Almond & Cacao Bars

Summer Berry & White
Chocolate Raw Mousse Cake

Carrot, Apple &
Orange Cake with
Cashew & Orange Icing

Chocolate Truffles

New York-Style Baked Coconut
& Vanilla "Cheesecake" with
Stewed Rhubarb

Rich Chocolate, Peanut
Butter & Raspberry Tart

Welsh Cakes with Whipped
"Cream" & Strawberries

MINT, CHOC CHIP & MATCHA ICE CREAM

Mint and choc chip has always been my favourite ice-cream flavour; I've included a little matcha in this recipe for the health benefits, vibrant colour and subtle taste it adds.

SERVES 6

1 x 400-ml (14-oz) can coconut milk

1 vanilla pod

handful of fresh mint leaves

140g (³/₄ cup) caster (superfine) sugar

2 tsp matcha powder

¹/₂ tsp xanthan gum

300ml (1¹/₂ cups) cashew Milk (see page 12)

140g (5oz) vegan dark chocolate, cut into small chunks

Heat the coconut milk in a saucepan. Split the vanilla pod down the middle and, using the back of a knife, scrape the seeds out of both sides. Add the seeds and pod to the saucepan, followed by the mint leaves and sugar. Simmer the mixture for 15 minutes until the flavours have infused, then pour into a mixing bowl and leave to cool.

Mix together the matcha, xanthan and cashew milk in a separate mixing bowl.

Once the mint-coconut milk mixture is cool, whisk it into the matcha-cashew mixture.

Cover with cling film (plastic wrap) and chill the mixture in the fridge to cool completely before pouring into an ice cream machine.

Before it starts to set in the machine, scatter in the chocolate. Churn the mix in the ice cream machine (according to the machine's instructions) until frozen, then transfer to a freezer-proof container and into the freezer.

Alternatively, if you don't have an ice cream machine, pour the mixture into a freezer-proof container and pop into the freezer. Mix it every hour with a spatula – do this around 5 times – adding the chocolate just before it sets.

Serve in bowls or ice cream cones. Store in a freezer set at -18°C (0°F).

RAW MANGO & VANILLA ICE CREAM

**Here's a healthier ice cream option;
it is sweetened only with natural sugar.**

SERVES 6

225g (1½ cups) raw cashew nuts,
soaked in water for at least 1 hour

320ml (1¼ cups) coconut milk

3 tbsp maple syrup

1 tsp vanilla bean paste

190g (1¼ cups) chopped mango

Drain the soaked cashew nuts,
add the nuts and the rest of the
ingredients to a powerful blender
and blitz until the mixture is super-
smooth. If you can't get rid of all
the lumps you will probably need
to add a little more coconut milk.

Once completely smooth, pour the
mixture into an ice cream machine
to churn until frozen (according
to the machine's instructions),
then transfer into a freezer-proof
container and into the freezer.

Alternatively, if you don't have
an ice cream machine, pour the
mixture into a freezer-proof
container and pop into the freezer.
Mix it every hour with a spatula
around 5–6 times.

Serve in bowls or ice cream cones.
Store in a freezer set at -18°C (0°F).

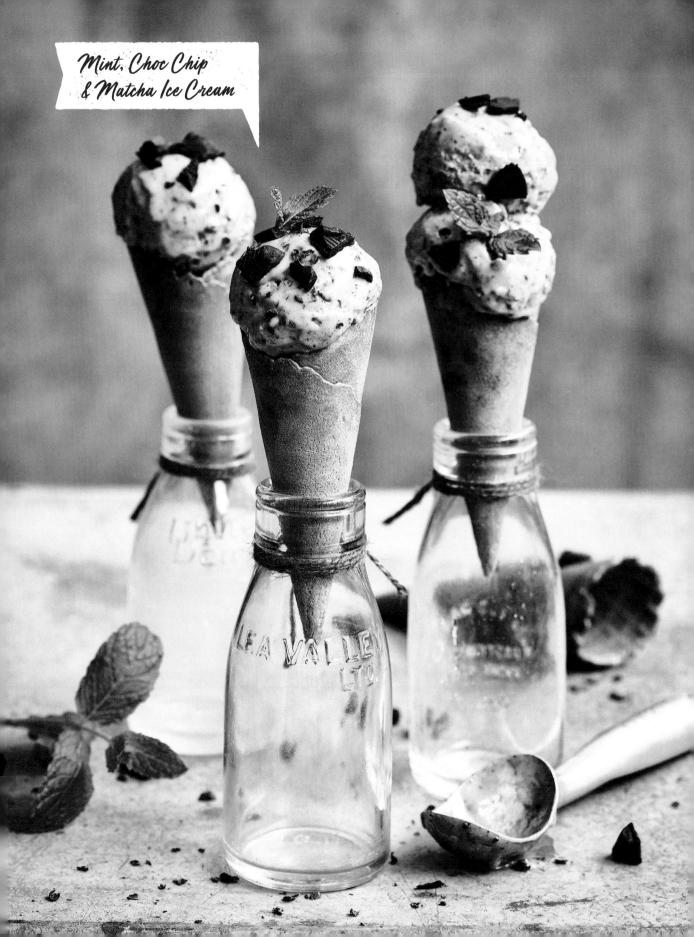

Mint, Choc Chip
& Matcha Ice Cream

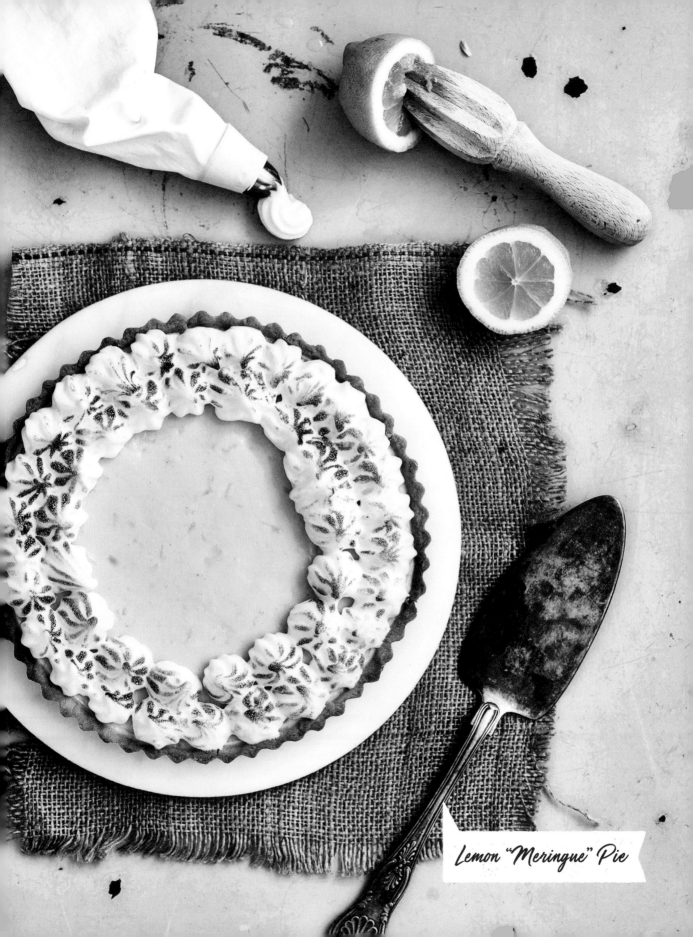

Lemon "Meringue" Pie

LEMON "MERINGUE" PIE

Light, creamy and, of course, lemony. After many attempts, I was over the moon when I successfully managed to veganize this classic dessert. The optional turmeric gives the filling a more intense yellow and doesn't alter the flavour at all.

SERVES 8–10

1 quantity Sweet Pastry
(see page 29)

1 x 400-ml (14-oz) can
coconut milk

2 tbsp lemon zest,
plus a little extra

juice of 2 lemons

280ml (1¼ cups) almond
Milk (see page 12)

4 heaped tbsp cornflour
(cornstarch)

5 tbsp unrefined caster
(superfine) sugar

½ tsp ground turmeric (optional)

235ml (1 cup) chickpea water –
"aquafaba" (this is just the liquid
drained from a can of chickpeas)

60g (½ cup) icing
(confectioner's) sugar

1 tsp vanilla extract

¼ tsp xanthan gum

First up, make the pastry following the recipe on page 29.

Preheat the oven to 180°C (350°F). Grease a 23-cm (9-inch) loose-bottom tart tin.

Remove your pastry from the fridge and roll out onto a sheet of greaseproof paper. Slide the pastry off the paper and into the tart tin to line it. Trim off any excess over-hanging pastry.

Cover with a piece of greaseproof paper, weigh down with baking beans, then blind-bake the pastry for 6 minutes.

Remove from the oven, carefully lift out the paper and beans, and return to the oven to bake for 6 minutes more, or until golden.

Once the pastry case is cooked, let it cool in the tin for 5 minutes before carefully removing and transferring to a wire rack to cool completely.

Now make the lemon custard filling: gently heat the coconut milk with the lemon zest and juice in a medium saucepan over a low heat.

Combine the almond milk, cornflour and caster sugar, and whisk until completely incorporated.

When the coconut milk is hot, add the almond milk and sugar mixture and whisk until the mixture starts to thicken. Add the turmeric if you want a bright yellow colour. Continue to whisk for 2 more minutes until the mixture is super-thick.

Carefully pour the lemon filling into the tart case and neatly spread it out using a stepped palette knife.

Place a piece of cling film (plastic wrap) directly over the lemon filling, making sure there are no air pockets. It's very important that the cling film makes direct contact with the filling as this stops a skin forming (which would crack and not look good).

Chill the tart in the fridge for at least 3 hours, until it's completely cold and set.

Just before serving, make your meringue.

Using an electric whisk, whisk the chickpea water, icing sugar, vanilla extract and xanthan gum together in a clean bowl, until you have stiff peaks.

Spoon or pipe the meringue onto your chilled tart. I lightly toast my meringue using a blow torch, but this is optional.

Sprinkle over lemon zest and serve.

CHOCOLATE FONDANTS

Simply heavenly: the ultimate vegan dessert. You can make these fondants gluten free if you replace the flour with a gluten-free self-raising blend.

MAKES 8

Wet:

240ml (1 cup) cashew Milk (see page 12)

2 tsp apple cider vinegar

2 tsp vanilla extract

4 tbsp Egg Replacement (see page 32)

115g (½ cup) vegan "butter"

Dry:

240g (2 cups) plain (all-purpose) flour

3 tbsp cacao powder

200g (1 cup) unrefined caster (granulated) sugar

3 tsp baking powder

¼ tsp salt

¼ tsp ground cinnamon

For the filling:

300g (2 cups) chopped vegan organic dark chocolate

240ml (1 cup) cashew Milk (see page 12)

¼ tsp Himalayan salt

To serve:

cherries

a little cacao powder

First up, make the chocolate filling. Tip the chocolate into a mixing bowl. Heat the milk with the salt, until piping hot, then pour over the chocolate and mix together until smooth and creamy. Place the bowl into the freezer to chill quickly.

Preheat the oven to 180°C (350°F). Grease 8 individual pudding moulds.

Heat all of the wet ingredients together in a small saucepan over a low heat, stirring until everything has melted and combined.

Combine the dry ingredients in a mixing bowl, then pour in the heated wet ingredients and stir until just combined.

Fill each pudding mould half full with the mixture, then place a tablespoonful of the chilled chocolate ganache into the middle of each. Fill the moulds with the rest of the fondant mixture, then give each mould a tap on the work surface to level them out.

Transfer to a baking tray, then bake for 12 minutes. Allow to cool slightly before turning the fondants out of the moulds.

Serve with cherries and a sprinkling of cacao powder.

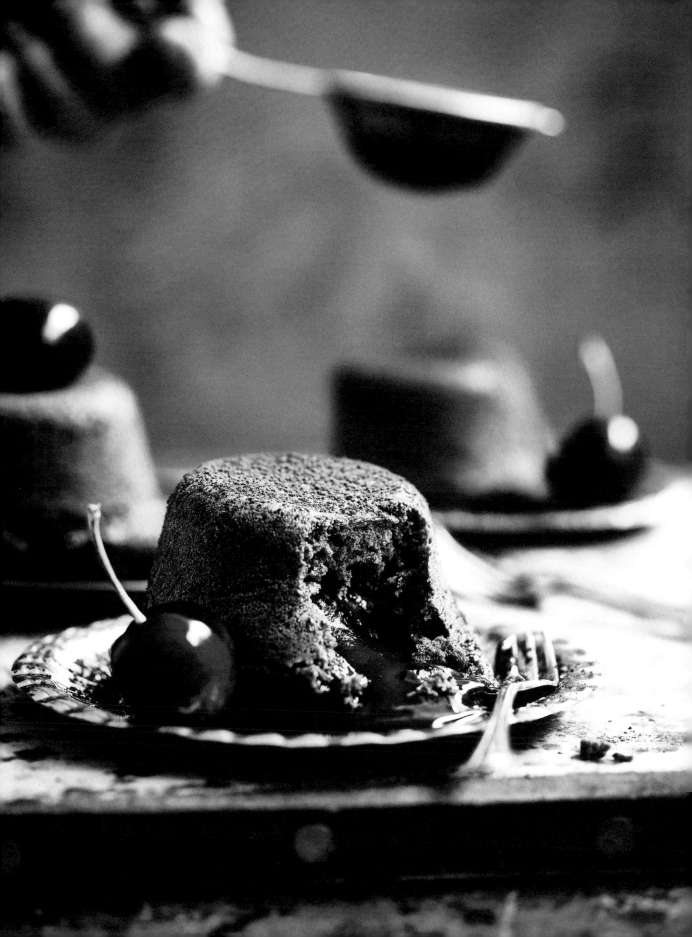

FANCY BAKED DOUGHNUTS

Definitely a once-in-a-while treat! I've included two of my favourite toppings but feel free to get adventurous and try making your own. You'll need a couple of 6-hole doughnut trays for this recipe.

MAKES 12 DOUGHNUTS

Wet:

240ml (1 cup) soy milk

110g (½ cup) vegan "butter"

4 tbsp Egg Replacement (see page 32)

2 tsp vanilla extract

Dry:

240g (2 cups) plain (all-purpose) flour

200g (1 cup) unrefined caster (granulated) sugar

2½ tsp baking powder

¼ tsp fine sea salt

¼ tsp ground cinnamon

¼ tsp grated nutmeg

Preheat the oven to 180°C (350°F). Grease 2 doughnut trays lightly with vegetable oil.

Heat all of the wet ingredients in a small saucepan over a low heat until everything has melted and mixed together. Remove from the heat.

Mix all of the dry ingredients together in a large mixing bowl. Make a well in the middle and pour in the wet mixture. Stir well until you have a thick batter.

Ladle batter into each doughnut ring. The neater you are, the more perfect your doughnuts will look, so clean off any drips.

Place the trays into the oven on the middle shelf to bake for 14 minutes, or until lightly golden.

Remove the doughnuts from the oven and allow to slightly cool for 5 minutes before turning them out of the trays. Apply one of the suggested toppings opposite, or alternatively just sprinkle with coconut sugar to serve.

CHOCOLATE, HONEYCOMB & STRAWBERRY TOPPING

FOR 6 DOUGHNUTS

4 tbsp golden syrup

200g (1 cup) unrefined caster (granulated) sugar

3 tsp bicarbonate of soda (baking soda)

120ml (1/2 cup) almond Milk (see page 12)

175g (1 cup) chopped vegan dark cooking chocolate

3 strawberries, halved

Grease and line a small baking tin with baking paper.

Melt the golden syrup and sugar together in a large saucepan over a low heat until amber coloured. Be very careful when making the honeycomb as melted sugar is extremely hot. Once you've reached the amber stage, turn the heat off and stir in the bicarbonate of soda as quickly as you can, until it dissolves and the mixture starts foaming.

Quickly and carefully scrape the mixture into the lined baking tin and put the honeycomb to one side to set hard. This should take around an hour. Break into pieces to serve.

For the chocolate topping, heat the milk in a small saucepan until piping hot. Tip the chocolate into a mixing bowl. Pour the hot milk over the chocolate, leave for a couple of minutes, then stir until thick and creamy.

Dip your doughnuts into the chocolate then top with the honeycomb and a strawberry half.

PISTACHIO, MINT & CHERRY TOPPING

FOR 6 DOUGHNUTS

125g (1 cup) unrefined icing (confectioner's) sugar

2 tbsp almond Milk (see page 12)

1/4 tsp peppermint extract

1/4 tsp natural green food colouring

handful of shelled pistachio nuts, chopped

6 cherries

Mix together the icing sugar, milk, peppermint extract and food colouring in a bowl. Dip the doughnuts into the icing, then sprinkle over pistachios and pop a cherry in the middle.

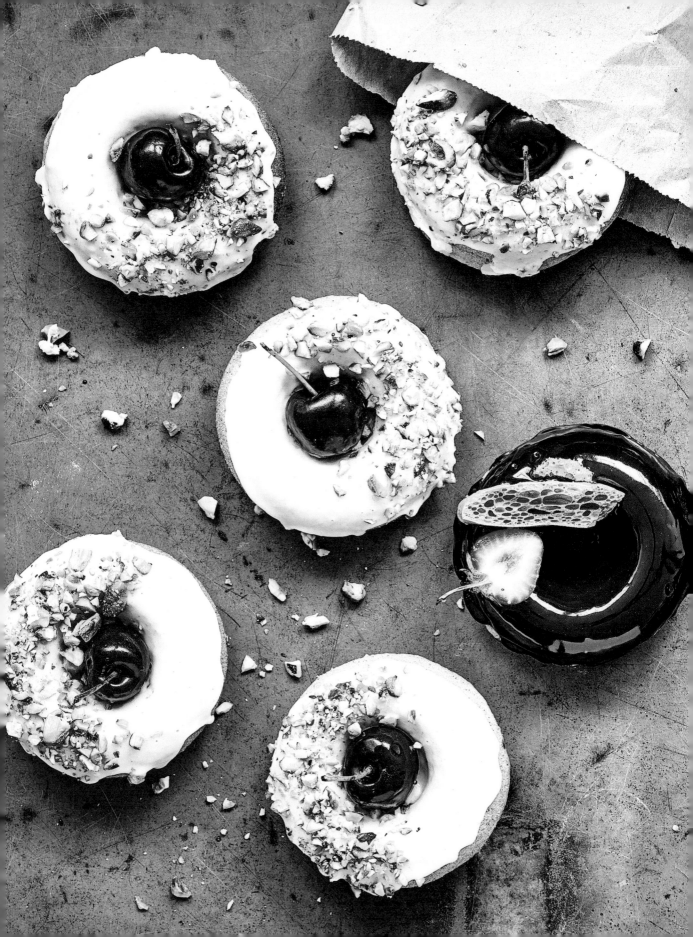

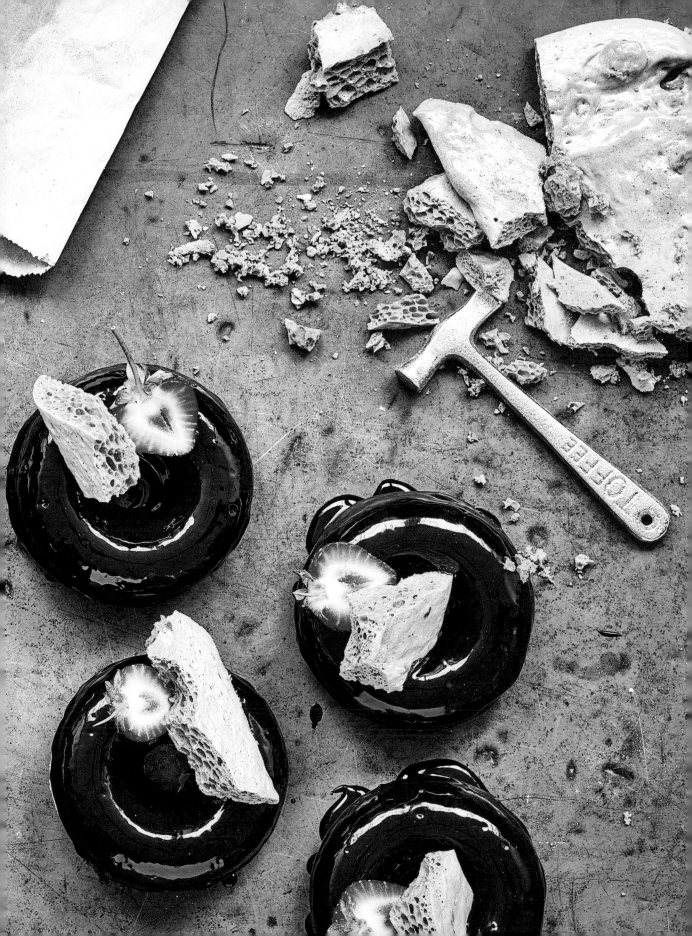

SALTED-CARAMEL PRETZEL, ALMOND & CACAO BARS

Rich and indulgent. These salted-caramel bars are 100% raw (without the pretzels) and only contain natural sugars, but they are definitely still a treat. Dates are a great energy food and are high in fibre, calcium and iron, plus so much more.

MAKES 12–14

For the almond "biscuit" layer:

70g (½ cup) macadamia nuts

40g (½ cup) coconut flakes

3 tbsp agave nectar

3 tbsp coconut oil

1 tbsp Peanut & Almond Butter (see page 33)

pinch Himalayan salt

170g (1½ cups) ground almonds

For the salted date caramel layer:

340g (2 cups) pitted Medjool dates

2 tbsp coconut oil

240ml (1 cup) almond Milk (see page 12)

120ml (½ cup) filtered water

1 tsp vanilla bean paste

¼ tsp Himalayan salt

For the "chocolate" coating:

5 tbsp coconut oil, melted

4 tbsp organic cacao powder

2 tbsp agave nectar

For the topping:

gluten-free pretzels, or flaked almonds (for 100% raw)

———————————————

Line a square, loose-bottom 20-cm (8-inch) baking tray with greaseproof paper.

First make the almond biscuit layer: blitz all of the ingredients, except the ground almonds, in the blender until the nuts and coconut are finely chopped. Add the ground almonds then pulse until fully incorporated. The mixture should be sticky.

Press the almond mixture into the base of the baking tray, making sure it's an even layer all over.

Pop the tray into the freezer and get on with the caramel layer.

Rinse out the blender. Blitz all the ingredients in the blender until the mixture is as smooth as possible.

Remove the tray from the freezer and spread the caramel layer over

the top evenly. Pop the tray back into the freezer to set for around 2 hours.

After the 2 hours, remove the tray from the freezer, carefully remove the bar from the tin, then cut it into 12–14 bars. Run your knife under hot water between each cut to make it easier.

Place the bars onto a baking tray and back into the freezer while you make the coating.

Mix the chocolate coating ingredients together in a small mixing bowl until smooth.

Remove the bars from the freezer and drizzle the coating over the top of each bar. Top each bar with a couple of pretzels or a sprinkling of flaked almonds. Serve straight away or store in the freezer for up to 2 months. Serve straight from the freezer.

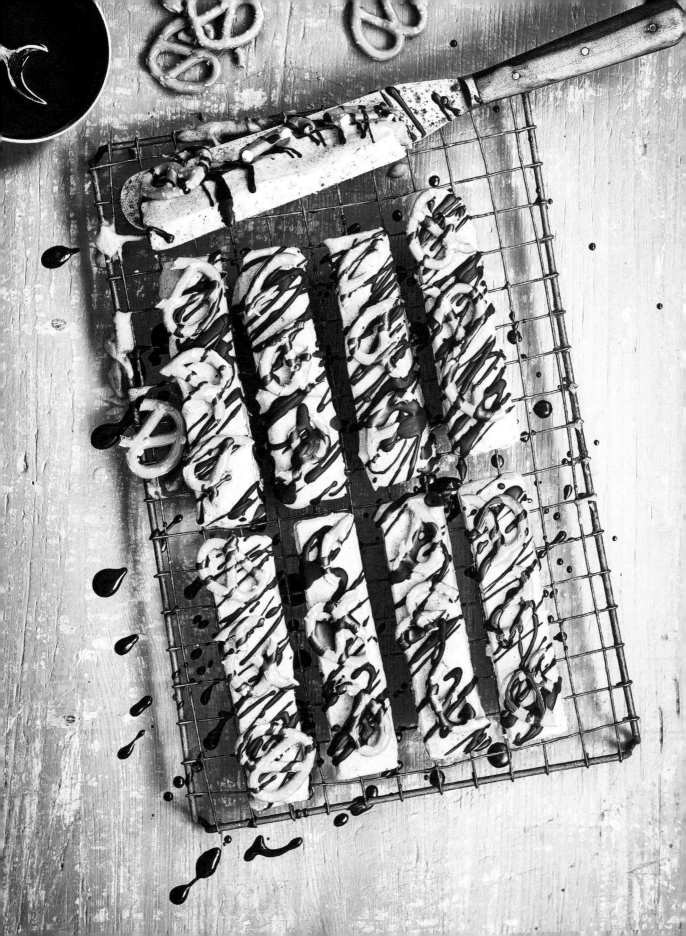

SUMMER BERRY & WHITE CHOCOLATE RAW MOUSSE CAKE

Bursting with berries, this raw, gluten-free "cheesecake" is surprisingly light and creamy. My homemade raw white chocolate works so well with it, too. The cake can be stored in the freezer for a few weeks until ready to serve. I like to make individual cakes, but you can make one large cake if you prefer.

SERVES 6–8, OR MAKES 6–8 SMALL CAKES

For the base:

260g (1½ cups) pitted dates

120g (1 cup) ground almonds

2 tbsp coconut oil

1 tbsp vanilla extract

For the filling:

340g (2½ cups) raw cashew nuts, soaked in water for at least 1 hour

150g (¾ cup) coconut oil, melted

60ml (¼ cup) almond Milk (see page 12)

1 x 400-ml (14-oz) can coconut milk

5 tbsp agave nectar

2 tsp vanilla extract

260g (1½ cups) frozen mixed berries

Toppings:

Raw White Raspberry Chocolate (see page 201)

fresh berries

fresh mint leaves

If making individual cakes, line a baking tray with greaseproof paper and place six or eight 8-cm (3-inch) stainless steel rings on the tray. Make enough room in your freezer for the tray. Alternatively, line a 23-cm (9-inch) loose-bottom cake tin with greaseproof paper.

First up, make the base. Add all of the ingredients to a blender and blitz until the mixture is smooth and starts to combine.

Spoon the mixture into your moulds or cake tin to around 1cm (⅓ inch) deep. Chill in the freezer while you make the filling.

Clean out the blender, then add the drained soaked cashew nuts and blitz until extra fine. Add the remaining filling ingredients, except the berries, and blitz until you have a thick creamy mixture. Make sure it's completely smooth, then scrape into a large bowl.

Clean out the blender, then add the berries and blend until smooth. Place a sieve over the bowl full of the filling mix and pass the berry

mixture through to remove any of the seeds. Lightly stir the berry mix into the filling to create a ripple effect.

Pour this mixture into the moulds or cake tin and place in the freezer for a couple of hours to set through.

Remove the cakes from the freezer 20 minutes before serving to give you time to decorate them and for them to soften slightly – they will be very hard if you try eating them straight from the freezer!

If you used ring moulds, pour boiling water over a tea towel and wrap it around each ring when you bring the cakes out of the freezer. This will loosen the edges and make it easier to release them.

Serve the cheesecake with shards of Raw White Raspberry Chocolate, fresh berries and a few mint leaves.

SWEET TALKING

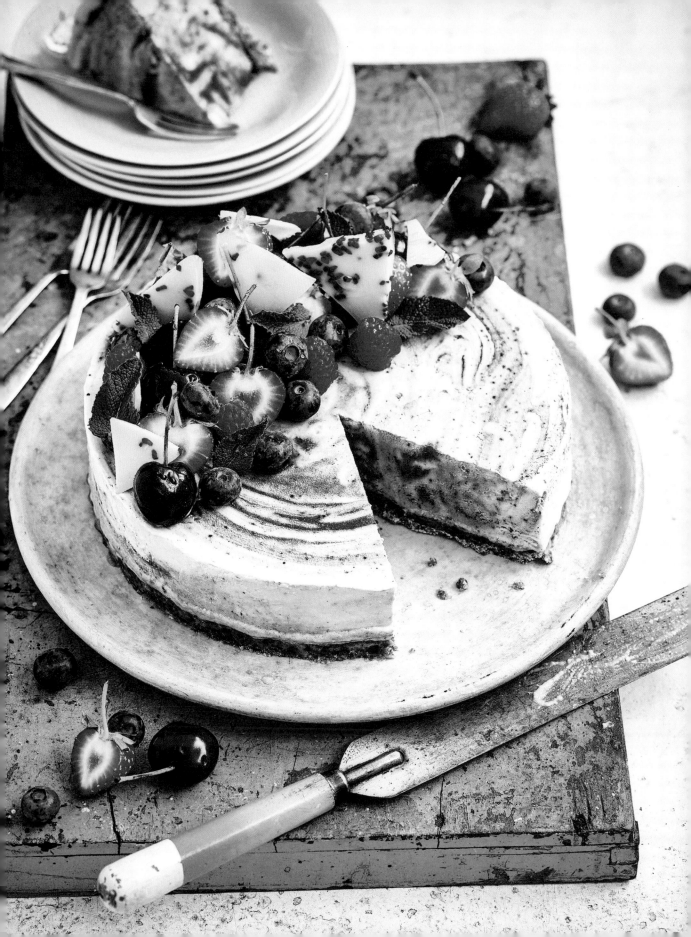

CARROT, APPLE & ORANGE CAKE WITH CASHEW & ORANGE ICING

I love simple rustic cakes like this. This one contains natural sugars and instead of the usual sugar-rich icing I've opted for a creamy nut-based icing which works beautifully. You can easily swap the flour for a gluten-free mix, too.

SERVES 12–14

240g (2 cups) self-raising flour

2 tsp baking powder (baking soda)

¼ tsp sea salt

1 tsp ground cinnamon

¼ tsp grated nutmeg

170g (1 cup) coconut sugar

125g (1 cup) walnuts, chopped

3 carrots, grated

1 apple, peeled and grated

zest of 1 orange

1 tsp vanilla extract

1 tbsp apple cider vinegar

80ml (⅓ cup) vegetable oil

240ml (1 cup) almond Milk (see page 12)

1 tbsp Egg Replacement (see page 32)

For the cashew & orange icing:

100g (1 cup) cashew nuts, soaked in water for 1 hour

60ml (¼ cup) cashew Milk (see page 12)

3 tbsp coconut oil, melted

juice and zest of ½ orange

3 tbsp maple syrup

1 tsp vanilla extract

Suggested toppings:

Dried Oranges (see opposite)

physalis

walnuts

Preheat the oven to 180°C (350°F). Grease and line a loose-bottom 25-cm (10-inch) cake tin.

Combine all of the dry ingredients in a large mixing bowl, then stir in the carrot, apple and orange. Add all the remaining cake ingredients and stir well to combine.

Pour the mixture into your lined cake tin and bake for 35 minutes. If you're unsure whether the cake is fully cooked, poke a metal skewer into the centre – if it comes out clean, it's cooked. If not, pop the cake back into the oven for a few minutes longer.

Let the cake rest and slightly cool before removing from the cake tin and cooling completely on a wire rack.

While the cake is cooling, make the icing. Drain away the soaking water from the nuts and add them to a blender with all of the other icing ingredients. Blitz until the icing is super-smooth, scrape into a bowl, cover with cling film (plastic wrap), then chill in the fridge for about 20 minutes before topping your cake.

When you're ready to serve, remove the icing from the fridge and use a palette knife to smooth the icing over the top of the cake. Top with dried oranges, walnuts and physalis, if using.

RAW WHITE
RASPBERRY CHOCOLATE

220g (1 cup) cacao butter, finely chopped

105g (½ cup) coconut oil

4 tbsp coconut sugar

2 tsp vanilla extract

3 tbsp freeze-dried raspberry bits

Line a medium baking tray with greaseproof paper.

Melt the cacao butter in a bowl over some simmering water, stirring often. Once melted, stir in the coconut oil until melted. Whisk in the sugar and vanilla and remove the bowl from the heat.

Allow it to cool slightly and thicken before stirring in the raspberry bits, then pour the mix into the lined baking tray and pop into the freezer to set firm.

DRIED ORANGES

1 orange, preferably unwaxed

1 tsp agave nectar

Preheat the oven to 110°C (230°F).

Slice the orange as thinly as possible and lay the slices in a single layer on a baking tray lined with greaseproof paper. Brush over a little agave nectar.

Bake for about 30 minutes. Keep checking them and remove as soon as they're looking dry.

Cool on the tray before peeling off the paper and using straight away, or you can store them in an airtight container for up to 3 days.

CHOCOLATE TRUFFLES

I used to make truffles often when I worked in commercial kitchens. We would make loads of different flavours and temper the chocolate. Tempering chocolate keeps it smooth and glossy, and adds a satisfying snap when you bite into it. I have a quick, cheat's way to do this without using a thermometer.

MAKES APPROXIMATELY 20

For the chocolate ganache filling:

480ml (2 cups) almond Milk (see page 12)

3 tbsp unrefined caster (granulated) sugar

1 tsp vanilla extract

700g (4 cups) finely chopped vegan dark chocolate

For the quick, tempered chocolate:

525g (3 cups) finely chopped vegan dark chocolate

Coatings:

75g (½ cup) hazelnuts, chopped

freeze-dried raspberry bits

cacao powder

Himalayan salt

First up, make the chocolate ganache filling. Heat the milk, sugar and vanilla extract in a small saucepan over a low heat.

Add the chocolate to a mixing bowl. Once the milk mixture is piping hot, pour it over the chocolate. Stir until there are no lumps and it's thick and creamy.

Pour the chocolate ganache into a shallow plastic container. (This makes it easier when forming into truffles.) Cover with cling film (plastic wrap) and chill in the fridge to set for around 2 hours.

Line a baking tray with greaseproof paper.

Once the chocolate ganache has set, it's time to ball it up into truffles. I use a melon baller for this to achieve uniform balls and I dip the baller into hot water before scooping out each ball. If you haven't got a melon baller, use a teaspoon to scoop the ganache, and your hands to form it into balls. (This can get messy!)

Place the ganache balls onto the lined baking tray as you go, then pop the tray into the fridge for them to firm up.

Meanwhile, prepare the quick, tempered chocolate and coatings.

Grab yourself a small saucepan and a medium-sized mixing bowl and make sure the bowl fits on top of the saucepan snugly.

Pour boiling water into the saucepan until half full and set over a medium heat. Place half of the chocolate into the bowl, sit the bowl on top of the saucepan, making sure the water isn't touching it, then turn the heat off.

Using a spatula, mix the chocolate until it's melted, and test with your finger to see if it's hot. Once it is hot, add half of the remaining chocolate and stir until melted. When it gets hot again, add the final quarter of chocolate and mix until fully melted.

Remove the ganache balls from the fridge. Put the chopped hazelnuts into a shallow bowl and get the other coatings ready.

Line a baking tray with greaseproof paper.

Using a fork, individually dip each ganache ball into the glossy melted chocolate.

For hazelnut truffles, go from the melted chocolate straight into the chopped hazelnuts. Then use your hands to roll and cover them with the nuts.

For the other coatings, place the truffles onto the tray and sprinkle with the raspberry bits, cacao powder or salt.

Place the coated truffles into the fridge to set firm for at least 1 hour before serving.

RAW CHOCOLATE ORANGE & PISTACHIO TRUFFLES

These raw truffles are not only indulgent, they give you a good energy and fibre boost.

300g (2 cups) pitted Medjool dates

4 tbsp raw cacao powder

zest of 1 orange

2 tbsp fresh orange juice

pinch sea salt

chopped pistachio nuts, to coat

Add all the ingredients to a food processor, except the pistachio nuts, and blitz until the mixture turns into a paste.

Lightly wet your hands and roll around 1 tablespoon of the paste into a ball. Repeat until you've rolled up all the mixture, then individually coat each ball in pistachio crumbs.

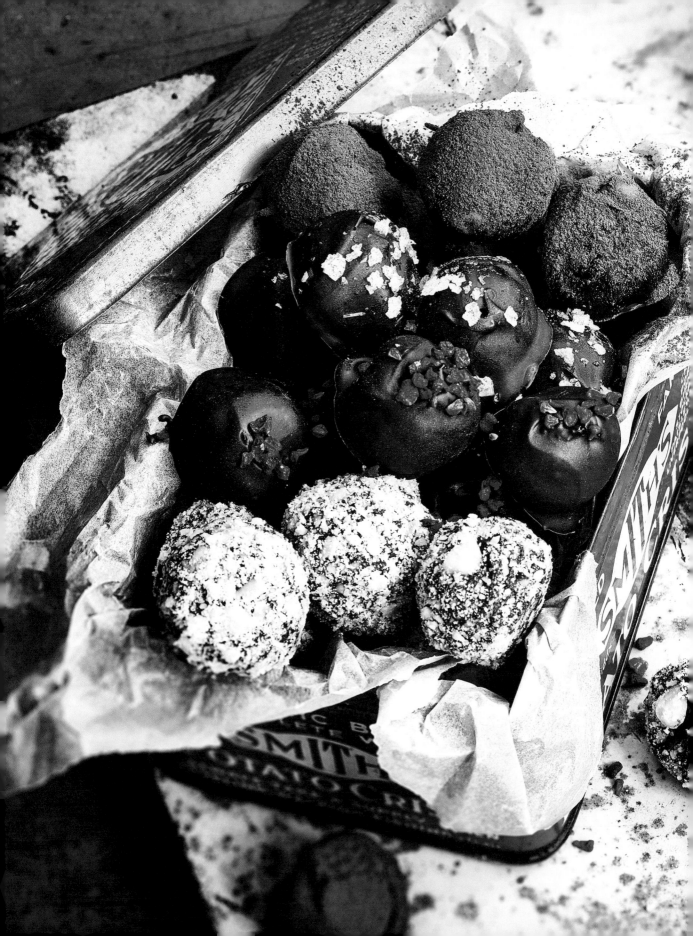

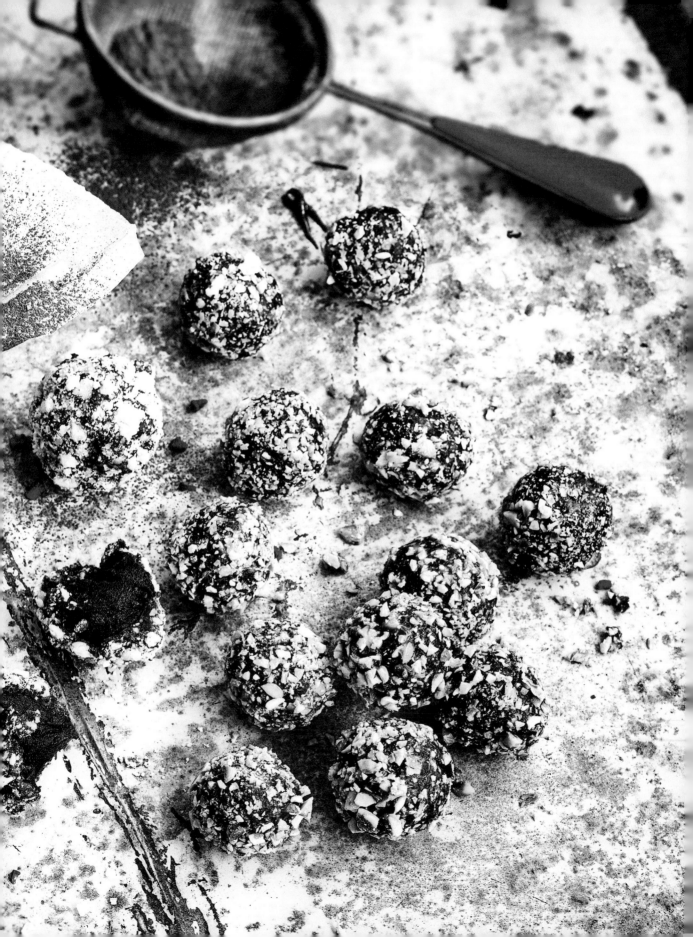

NEW YORK-STYLE BAKED COCONUT & VANILLA "CHEESECAKE" WITH STEWED RHUBARB

Here's another dessert I was thrilled about when I managed to veganize it – baked cheesecake was my favourite dessert before going vegan. I use shop-bought, coconut-based vegan "cream cheese" in the mix and caramel Biscoff biscuits for the base.

SERVES 10–12

fresh mint, to decorate

For the base:

300g (10½oz) Lotus Biscoff biscuits (cookies)

160g (⅔ cup) vegan "butter", melted

3 tbsp coconut oil, melted

For the filling:

65g (½ cup) almond flour

360g (1⅓ cups) vegan "cream cheese"

1 x 400-ml (14-oz) can coconut milk

200g (1 cup) unrefined caster (granulated) sugar

5 tbsp plain (all-purpose) flour

3 tbsp cornflour (cornstarch)

2 tsp vanilla extract

For the stewed rhubarb:

4 sticks of rhubarb, chopped

juice and zest of 1 orange

120ml (½ cup) water

4 tbsp agave nectar

Preheat the oven to 170°C (340°F). Lightly grease a loose-bottom cake tin approximately 23cm (9 inches) in diameter and 7.5–10cm (3–4 inches) deep.

First make the base. Blitz the Biscoff biscuits in a blender until they are a fine crumb. Keep blending and add the butter and coconut oil. Tip the biscuit mixture into the greased cake tin and use a spoon to press the mixture to form an even biscuit layer in the base and up the sides. Pop the tin into the fridge until needed.

Clean out the blender. Put the almond flour in the blender with the cream cheese and coconut milk. Blend until the mixture is super-smooth. Add the sugar, flour and cornflour and lightly blend until they are well incorporated. Finally, add the vanilla extract to taste and pulse to mix.

Remove the base from the fridge, pour in the filling and smooth the top, making sure it's level.

Fill a deep baking tray with warm water around 2.5cm (1 inch) high, then place the cake tin into it. NB If you are using a cake tin that isn't sealed you must wrap the bottom of the tin with foil to stop any water getting into the cake.

Carefully transfer the tray to the middle shelf of the oven to bake for 1 hour.

After 1 hour of cooking, carefully remove the tray from the oven and leave to cool for 1 hour before removing the cake from the tray. Wipe the bottom dry and chill in the fridge to set through for at least 3 hours.

Meanwhile, make the stewed rhubarb. Simply heat the chopped rhubarb in a saucepan with the rest of the ingredients and simmer over a low heat for 8–10 minutes, or until the rhubarb is tender.

Once the cake has chilled right through, carefully release it from the cake tin. Use a hot knife to cut slices and serve with the warm stewed rhubarb. Decorate with fresh mint.

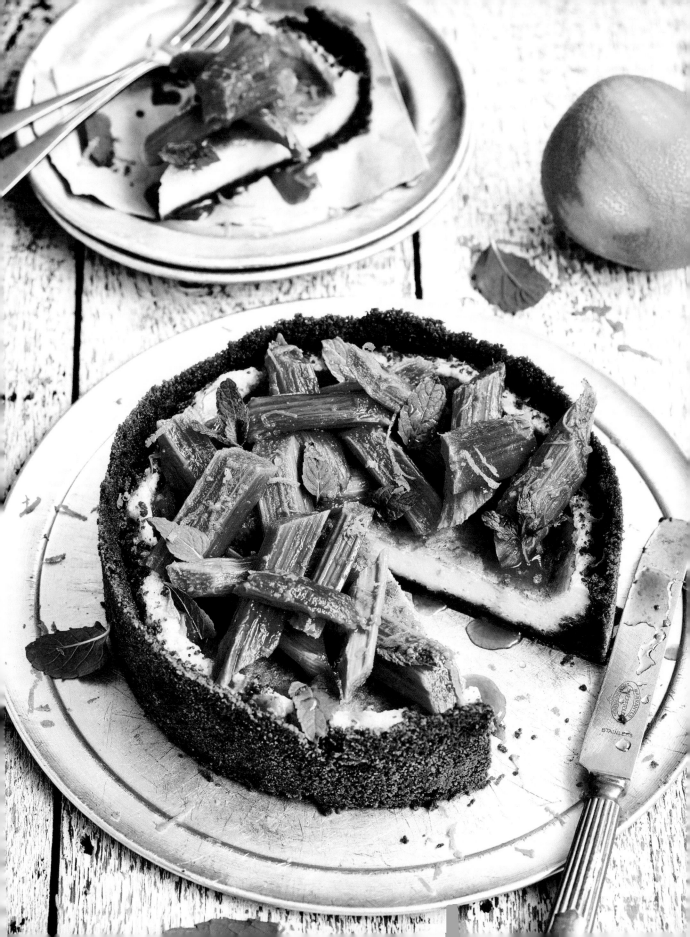

RICH CHOCOLATE, PEANUT BUTTER & RASPBERRY TART

This dessert is truly decadent as the chocolate filling is so rich and creamy. Adding the peanut butter and raspberry element creates an almost nostalgic taste of peanut butter and jam sandwiches.

SERVES 8–10

1 quantity Sweet Pastry
(see page 29) with 2 tbsp
cacao powder added

250g (2 cups) fresh raspberries

1 tbsp icing (confectioner's) sugar

295ml (1¼ cups) almond
Milk (see page 12)

2 tbsp smooth peanut butter

2 tbsp agave nectar

1 vanilla pod

400g (2½ cups) finely chopped
vegan dark chocolate

For the peanut brittle:

225g (1½ cups) raw peanuts

400g (2 cups) unrefined
caster (granulated) sugar

2 tbsp water

To garnish:

sprinkling of raw cacao powder

Preheat the oven to 180°C (350°F) and grease a 23-cm (9-inch) loose-bottom tart tin. Make the pastry following the recipe on page 29, adding the cacao.

Remove your pastry from the fridge and roll out onto a sheet of greaseproof paper. Slide the pastry off the paper and into the tart tin to line it. Trim off any excess over-hanging pastry. Cover with a piece of greaseproof paper, weigh down with baking beans, then blind-bake the pastry for 6 minutes. Remove from the oven, lift out the paper and beans, and return to the oven to bake for 6 minutes more, or until golden.

Once the pastry case is cooked, let it cool in the tin for 5 minutes, then carefully remove and transfer to a wire rack to cool completely.

The first element of the filling is the raspberry layer. Mash the raspberries and icing sugar in a mixing bowl using a fork. Spoon the raspberry mixture into a sieve over a jug to let some of the excess liquid drain out, so that it doesn't spoil the crispness of the pastry.

Spread the raspberry mixture evenly in the bottom of the pastry case.

Pour the milk into a small saucepan and add the peanut butter and agave. Split the vanilla pod in half lengthways with a small knife, using the back of the knife to scrape out the seeds from both halves. Add the seeds and the vanilla pod to the milk. Heat the saucepan over a low heat and whisk until the mixture is well incorporated and piping hot.

Tip the chopped chocolate into a mixing bowl. Carefully remove the vanilla pod from the hot milk and peanut mixture before pouring it over the chocolate. Use a spatula to mix until all the chocolate has melted and the filling is thick and creamy. (Try not to eat any!)

Carefully pour the chocolate filling into the pastry case over the raspberries until just below the top of the pastry edge, then transfer to the fridge to chill for at least 2 hours.

To make the peanut brittle, spread the peanuts out on a baking tray lined with greaseproof paper.

Melt the sugar and water in a small saucepan over a medium heat until it turns a golden amber colour. This should take around 10 minutes.

Quickly and carefully pour the melted sugar over the peanuts, then leave the tray somewhere safe to cool for around 1 hour. Please be very careful when making the brittle as the sugar gets extremely hot. When the brittle is cold, use a rolling pin to break up into shards.

To serve, cut the tart using a hot knife and serve with a shard of peanut brittle.

WELSH CAKES WITH WHIPPED "CREAM" & STRAWBERRIES

Well, I am Welsh after all... I have used and tinkered with this recipe for years, but altered it to be vegan just a couple of years ago. It works! I just love being Welsh and these Welsh cakes!

MAKES 12–14 CAKES

210g (1³/₄ cups) plain (all-purpose) flour

100g (¹/₂ cup) unrefined caster (granulated) sugar, plus extra for coating

75g (²/₃ cup) mixed currants

1 tsp baking powder

¹/₂ tsp ground cinnamon

pinch grated nutmeg

pinch salt

125g (¹/₂ cup) vegan "butter"

120ml (¹/₂ cup) almond Milk (see page 12)

a little coconut oil

For the whipped "cream":

400g (14oz) coconut cream

2 tbsp icing (confectioner's) sugar

1 tsp vanilla extract

To serve:

fresh strawberries

Combine all the dry ingredients in a large mixing bowl. Add the vegan butter and rub into the flour mixture with your fingers to form a breadcrumb-like consistency. Pour in enough milk to bind the mix into a dough.

Tip the dough out onto a floured work surface and roll to the thickness of your little finger.

Using a 5-cm (2-inch) cutter, cut the dough into discs.

Preheat a heavy-based skillet over a low heat. Rub a tiny bit of coconut oil into the pan then cook a few cakes at a time for 3 minutes on each side, until golden.

Sprinkle over the additional sugar while the cakes are still hot.

To make the whipped cream, put the coconut cream into a bowl with the sugar and vanilla extract, and whisk until thick and creamy.

Serve the Welsh cakes with a dollop of cream and a few fresh strawberries.

HEALTH POTIONS

Here's a collection of my favourite juices and shakes!
They're great for giving me an energy boost before a
long day of cooking, or even after a big workout when
a hit of added protein is needed. Feel free to add
different fruits or vegetables to your blends.

PINEAPPLE KICK

SERVES 2–3

600g (2 cups) peeled
and cubed pineapple

2 handfuls of kale,
shredded and washed

1 tsp chopped fresh jalapeño chilli

handful of fresh mint

approximately 12-cm
(5-inch) piece of cucumber

Process everything through a
juicer, then pour into glasses and
serve. I like to use refrigerated
pineapple and cucumber so that
my juice is cold.

If you don't have a juicer, use
a blender and strain the juice
through a fine sieve into a jug.

GREEN BLAST SMOOTHIE

SERVES 2–3

1 ripe avocado, peeled, de-stoned and cubed

handful of kale, shredded and washed

handful of spinach, washed

1 kiwi, chopped

1 tbsp wheatgrass powder

1 tbsp agave nectar

juice of $\frac{1}{2}$ lime

700ml (3 cups) coconut water

Blend everything together in a high-speed blender until smooth, then pour into glasses and serve with ice.

SUNSHINE ORANGE

SERVES 2–3

6 organic carrots, peeled

2 blood oranges, peeled

thumb-sized piece of fresh ginger, peeled

1.5-cm ($\frac{1}{2}$-in) piece of turmeric root, peeled

Process everything through a juicer, then pour into glasses and serve. I like to use refrigerated carrots and oranges so that my juice is cold.

If you don't have a juicer, use a blender and strain the juice through a fine sieve into a jug.

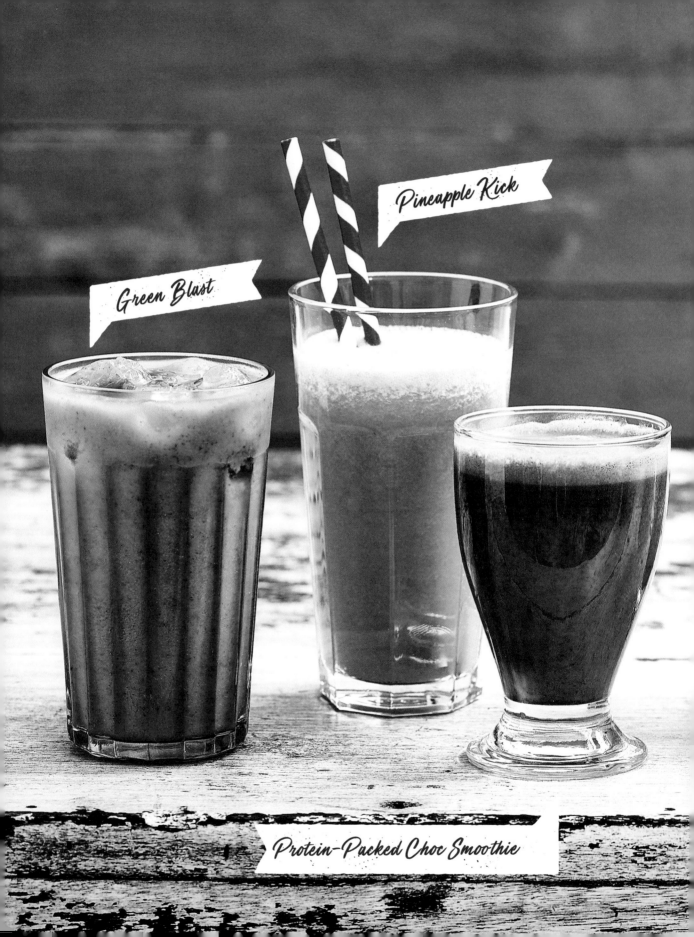

Green Blast

Pineapple Kick

Protein-Packed Choc Smoothie

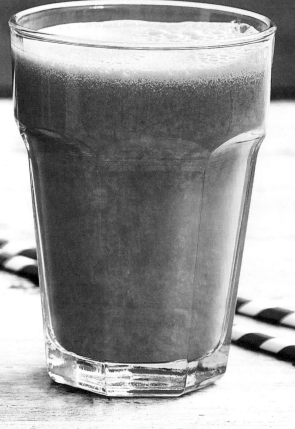

Sunshine Orange

The Purp

PROTEIN-PACKED CHOC SMOOTHIE

SERVES 2–3

1 frozen banana

50g ($\frac{1}{2}$ cup) fresh blueberries

3 tbsp raw cacao paste

2 tbsp cacao powder

2 tbsp shelled hemp seeds

2 tbsp goji berries

1 tbsp agave nectar

3 tbsp rolled oats

600ml ($2\frac{1}{2}$ cups) cashew Milk (see page 12)

Optional toppings:

whipped coconut cream

cacao nibs

grated raw chocolate

Process all the ingredients in a blender, then pour into glasses and serve. If the smoothie is slightly too thick, add more milk. Top with whipped coconut cream, cacao nibs and raw chocolate shavings.

THE PURP

SERVES 2–3

1 organic beetroot (beet), peeled

125g (1 cup) fresh blackberries

1 apple

approximately 12-cm (5-inch) piece of cucumber

2 handfuls of spinach, washed

1 stick of celery

Process all the ingredients through a juicer, then pour into glasses and serve. I like to use refrigerated fruit and veg so that my juice is cold.

If you don't have a juicer, use a blender and strain the juice through a fine sieve into a jug.

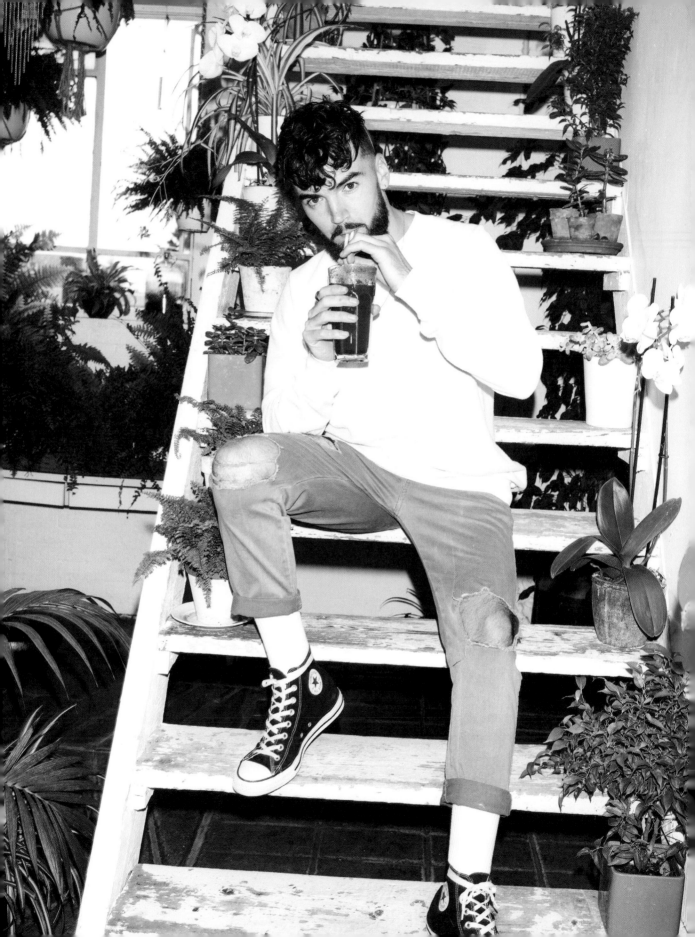

INDEX

ACKNOWLEDGMENTS

I would like to thank the following people who have helped make my debut cookbook possible, and supported me from the very beginning.

This could not have happened without the incredible team at Quadrille Publishing – a special thank you to Helen Lewis & Céline Hughes. To Zoe Ross for making my dream of having a cookbook a reality. To Simon Smith, the genius who shot all the pictures and taught me loads about food photography in the process. To my school friend Joe Horner who did an incredible job assisting me throughout the shoot, and the talented Jo Ormiston for designing the book.

To my incredible parents, Doug & Juliet, for believing in me right from the start and letting me take over their kitchen most days.

To my girlfriend Giorgia Sugarman for always being so supportive.

Thanks to the great brands who have worked with me from the start of @avantgardevegan. Special thank you to Ninja Kitchen UK.

Thank you to the crews that have filmed and edited my YouTube videos since I launched my channel.

To my good friend Mark Parry, one of the first chefs I worked with who I really looked up to, along with Matt Larsen.

A HUGE thank you to all my incredible social media followers and YouTube subscribers – without your support, this book would not exist.

Gaz

First published in 2018 by Quadrille,
an imprint of Hardie Grant Publishing

Quadrille
52-54 Southwark Street
London, SE1 1UN
quadrille.com

Cataloguing in Publication Data: a catalogue record for
this book is available from the British Library.

ISBN 978 1 78713 124 8

Printed and bound in China

Reprinted in 2017
10 9 8 7 6 5 4 3 2

Publishing director: Sarah Lavelle
Creative director: Helen Lewis
Commissioning editor: Céline Hughes
Art direction and design: Jo Ormiston
Design assistants: Emily Lapworth and Gemma Hayden
Food photography: Simon Smith
Portrait photography: Adam Laycock
Endpaper photography: Gaz Oakley
Prop styling: Luis Peral, with Gaz Oakley
Food styling: Gaz Oakley
Production manager: Stephen Lang
Production director: Vincent Smith

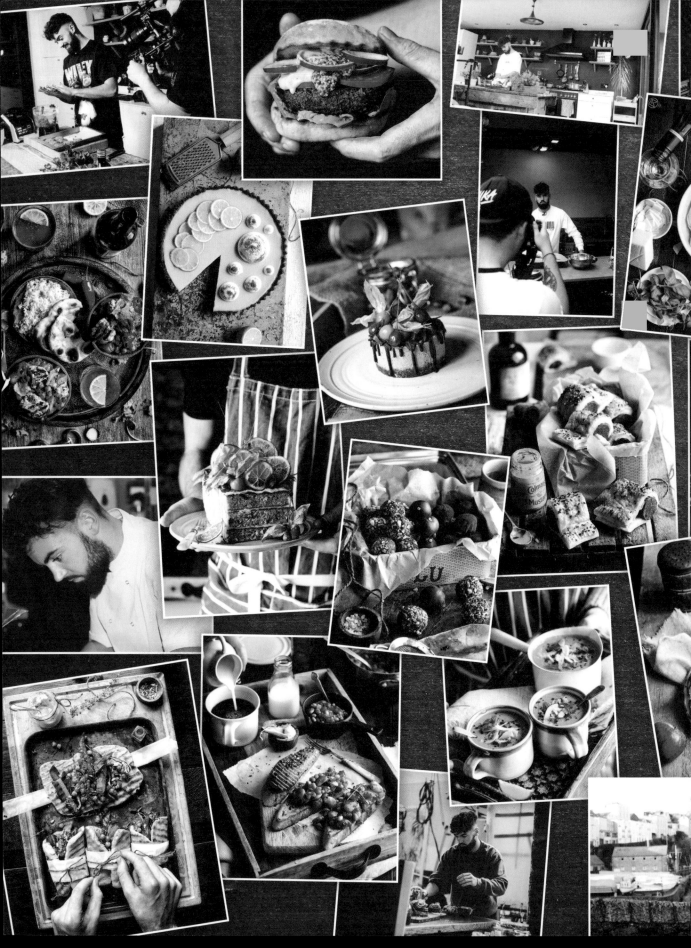